Clinicians' Guides to Radionuclide Hybrid Imaging

PET/CT

Series Editors

Jamshed B. Bomanji
London, UK

Gopinath Gnanasegaran
London, UK

Stefano Fanti
Bologna, Italy

Homer A. Macapinlac
Houston, Texas, USA

More information about this series at http://www.springer.com/series/13803

Kalevi Kairemo • Homer A. Macapinlac

Editors

Sodium Fluoride PET/CT in Clinical Use

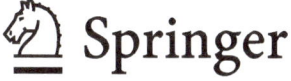 Springer

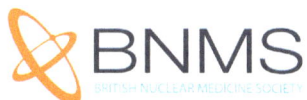

Editors
Kalevi Kairemo
Department of Nuclear Medicine
University of Texas MD Anderson Cancer
Center
Houston, TX
USA

Homer A. Macapinlac
Department of Nuclear Medicine
University of Texas MD Anderson Cancer
Center
Houston, TX
USA

ISSN 2367-2439　　　　　　ISSN 2367-2447　(electronic)
Clinicians' Guides to Radionuclide Hybrid Imaging - PET/CT
ISBN 978-3-030-23576-5　　　　ISBN 978-3-030-23577-2　(eBook)
https://doi.org/10.1007/978-3-030-23577-2

This Springer imprint is published by the registered company Springer Nature Switzerland AG
The registered company address is: Gewerbestrasse 11, 6330 Cham, Switzerland

PET/CT series is dedicated to Prof Ignac Fogelman, Dr Muriel Buxton-Thomas and Prof Ajit K Padhy

Foreword

Clear and concise clinical indications for PET/CT in the management of the oncology and non-oncology patient are presented in this series of 15 separate booklets.

The impact on better staging, tailored management and specific treatment of the patient with cancer has been achieved with the advent of this multimodality imaging technology. Early and accurate diagnosis will always pay, and clear information can be gathered with PET/CT on treatment responses. Prognostic information is gathered and can forward guide additional therapeutic options.

It is a fortunate coincidence that PET/CT was able to derive great benefit from radionuclide-labelled probes, which deliver good and often excellent target to non-target signals. Whilst labelled glucose remains the cornerstone for the clinical benefit achieved, a number of recent probes are definitely adding benefit. PET/CT is hence an evolving technology, extending its applications and indications. Significant advances in the instrumentation and data processing available have also contributed to this technology, which delivers high throughput and a wealth of data, with good patient tolerance and indeed patient and public acceptance. As an example, the role of PET/CT in the evaluation of cardiac disease is also covered, with emphasis on labelled rubidium and labelled glucose studies.

The novel probes of labelled choline; labelled peptides, such as DOTATATE; and, most recently, labelled PSMA (prostate-specific membrane antigen) have gained rapid clinical utility and acceptance, as significant PET/CT tools for the management of neuroendocrine disease and prostate cancer patients, notwithstanding all the advances achieved with other imaging modalities, such as MRI. Hence a chapter reviewing novel PET tracers forms a part of this series.

The oncological community has recognised the value of PET/CT and has delivered advanced diagnostic criteria for some of the most important indications for PET/CT. This includes the recent Deauville criteria for the classification of PET/CT patients with lymphoma—similar criteria are expected to develop for other malignancies, such as head and neck cancer, melanoma and pelvic malignancies. For completion, a separate section covers the role of PET/CT in radiotherapy planning, discussing the indications for planning biological tumour volumes in relevant cancers.

These booklets offer simple, rapid and concise guidelines on the utility of PET/CT in a range of oncological indications. They also deliver a rapid aide-memoire on the merits and appropriate indications for PET/CT in oncology.

London, UK   Peter J. Ell, FMedSci, DR HC, AΩA

Preface

Fluorine-18-labelled sodium fluoride [^{18}F-NaF] has a long history. Even though it is one of the easiest producible positron-labelled radiopharmaceuticals and its basic characteristics are known for several decades, it is still not as widely used as it should. ^{18}F-NaF-positron emission tomography (PET) can be used for assessing calcification processes in the body, i.e., bone formation, measuring turnover from hydroxyapatite to fluoroapatite.

The role of ^{18}F-NaF-PET and its capability of replacing bone scintigraphy (BS) has been used just for more than a decade in clinical routine even though it was discovered already in the 1960s. It is obvious that ^{18}F-NaF-PET has same indications as BS, but because it is more sensitive than BS, it may have limited indications in certain benign conditions, and new indications may occur. In malignant metastatic diseases, ^{18}F-NaF-PET has already shown its benefit. In the United States, there is a National PET Registry, and extensive data exists about its performance in cancer staging, restaging, follow-up, and response evaluation. ^{18}F-NaF-PET has an emerging diagnostic role in the calcified soft tissue metastases of primary bone tumors. Similarly, ^{18}F-NaF-PET can be applied to evaluate cardiovascular diseases, such as calcifications in heart valves and peripheral vascular disease.

In summary, there is a need for this kind of textbook, and it is the first one about ^{18}F-NaF-PET. It deals with all the abovementioned issues consisting of 11 chapters. Five of the chapters are related to oncology, four chapters deal with general aspects of ^{18}F-NaF-PET in benign skeletal conditions, and two chapters are related to cardiovascular diseases. We hope that this book will serve as a guide to referring colleagues, nuclear medicine physicians/radiologists, and aid clinicians participating in multidisciplinary meetings to describe the applications and limitations of ^{18}F-NaF-PET hybrid imaging (PET/CT).

Houston, TX, USA   Kalevi Kairemo
Houston, TX, USA   Homer A. Macapinlac

Acknowledgements

The series co-ordinators and editors would like to express sincere gratitude to the members of the British Nuclear Medicine Society, patients, teachers, colleagues, students, the industry and the BNMS Education Committee Members, for their continued support and inspiration.

Andy Bradley
Brent Drake
Francis Sundram
James Ballinger
Parthiban Arumugam
Rizwan Syed
Sai Han
Vineet Prakash

Contents

About the Authors

Kalevi Kairemo graduated with an MSc (Eng) degree from Helsinki University of Technology in 1980 before undertaking medical training (MD, PhD) at the University of Helsinki, Finland. He subsequently completed specialist training in Clinical Chemistry, Nuclear Medicine, and Clinical Pharmacology at Helsinki University Central Hospital (HUCH), followed by a research fellowship at Memorial Sloan-Kettering Cancer Center in New York (1989–1993). He has held posts as Professor of Clinical Chemistry at the Norwegian University of Science and Technology (1998–1999), Professor of Nuclear Medicine at Uppsala University Hospital in Sweden (2001–2005), and as Head of the Nuclear Medicine Division, Department of Oncology at HUCH (2004–2009). From 2009 to 2018, he was Chief of Nuclear Medicine and Molecular Radiotherapy at the Docrates Cancer Center in Helsinki. Since 2015 he has also been a Visiting Professor (Nuclear Medicine) at the University of Texas MD Anderson Cancer Center. Besides holding a few patents, he has published more than 200 original articles in peer-reviewed journals. In 2012, he received the Lifetime Achievement Award from the World Association of Radiopharmaceutical and Molecular Therapy.

Homer A. Macapinlac is the James E. Anderson Distinguished Professor of Nuclear Medicine and Chair of the Department of Nuclear Medicine at the University of Texas MD Anderson Cancer Center in Houston, Texas. Dr. Macapinlac is certified by the American Board of Nuclear Medicine, with a Certificate of Added Qualification (CAQ) in Nuclear Cardiology. He was also elected as a fellow of the American College of Nuclear Physicians. Prior to coming to MD Anderson, he served as clinical director of the Laurent and Alberta Gershel Positron Emission Tomography Center of Memorial Sloan-Kettering Cancer Center, New York. Dr. Macapinlac is an active committee member of various groups and has served as past Chair of the Institute of Clinical PET. He was Chair of the Society of Nuclear Medicine PET Center of Excellence and received the SNM Distinguished Service Award for this role. Dr. Macapinlac is also an expert consultant to the IAEA and an International Visiting Professor for the Radiological Society of North America. He has 199 peer-reviewed publications with 11,751 citations and an h-index of 57.

Contributors

Ana Emília Brito Real Nuclear, Real Hospital Português de Beneficência em Pernambuco, Recife, Brazil

Marwa Daghem Centre for Cardiovascular Science, University of Edinburgh, Edinburgh, UK

Elba Etchebehere Division of Nuclear Medicine, University of Campinas (UNICAMP), Campinas, Brazil

Lesley Flynt Department of Nuclear Medicine, University of Texas MD Anderson Cancer Center, Houston, TX, USA

Xu Guofan Department of Nuclear Medicine, University of Texas MD Anderson Cancer Center, Houston, TX, USA

Jakub Kaczynski British Heart Foundation Department of Cardiovascular Sciences, Queens Medical Research Institute, University of Edinburgh, Edinburgh, UK

Kalevi Kairemo Department of Nuclear Medicine, University of Texas MD Anderson Cancer Center, Houston, TX, USA

Department of Nuclear Medicine and Molecular Radiotherapy, Docrates Cancer Center, Helsinki, Finland

Homer A. Macapinlac Department of Nuclear Medicine, University of Texas MD Anderson Cancer Center, Houston, TX, USA

David E. Newby British Heart Foundation Department of Cardiovascular Sciences, Queens Medical Research Institute, University of Edinburgh, Edinburgh, UK

Vivek Subbiah Department of Investigational Cancer Therapeutics (Phase I Clinical Trials Program), Unit 455, Division of Cancer Medicine, The University of Texas MD Anderson Cancer Center, Houston, TX, USA

Maaz B. J. Syed British Heart Foundation Department of Cardiovascular Sciences, Queens Medical Research Institute, University of Edinburgh, Edinburgh, UK

Guofan Xu Department of Nuclear Medicine, University of Texas MD Anderson Cancer Center, Houston, TX, USA

^{18}F Sodium Fluoride: Tracer and Technique

1

Lesley Flynt

Contents

1.1 Historical Perspective

The first images of the bones of the skeleton date back to the late 1890s when German physicist Wilhelm Röntgen produced the first plain film by projecting X-rays through his wife's hand to produce a picture of the hand bones on a photographic plate [1, 2]. We have come a long way since the 1890s.

Standard radiology procedures continue to use this method of imaging by producing pictures of the human body by sending radiation from outside of the body, to the inside.

Nuclear medicine imaging, on the other hand, produces pictures of the human body by gathering radiation coming from inside of the body, to the outside. Further, nuclear techniques look at activity within the body by using targeted radiotracers. That is, nuclear medicine images are for viewing active physiologic processes, rather than anatomy.

L. Flynt (✉)
Department of Nuclear Medicine, University of Texas MD Anderson Cancer Center, Houston, TX, USA
e-mail: LFlynt@mdanderson.org

© Springer Nature Switzerland AG 2020   1
K. Kairemo, H. A. Macapinlac (eds.), *Sodium Fluoride PET/CT in Clinical Use*,
Clinicians' Guides to Radionuclide Hybrid Imaging,
https://doi.org/10.1007/978-3-030-23577-2_1

One of the first targeted radiotracers to be developed was Sodium 18-Fluoride (NaF). It was first discovered in the 1960s as a dedicated imaging agent of activity in the bony skeleton from the inside, out, and for the first time, allowed scientists and physicians the ability to visualize radiotracer distribution, or osteoblastic activity, in the bones of the human body [3].

It was during that time that nuclear imaging was performed using the Rectilinear Scanner which was invented by Benedict Cassen in 1949 [4, 5], specifically for the detection of radioactivity from the body, for medical use. This scanner had the capability to image a wide range of photon energies; however, it was quickly replaced by the gamma camera, or Anger camera, invented by Hal O. Anger in 1957 [5, 6]. The gamma camera produced images which were far superior to those of the Rectilinear Scanner; however, a limitation of the conventional gamma camera was the inability to image moderately high energy radionuclides. NaF has a moderately high energy [3, 5, 7–9].

To add to the decline of the use of NaF was the development of the table-top Molybdenum-99/Technetium-99 (^{99}Mo/^{99m}Tc) generator out of Brookhaven Labs in 1958 [10–12]. This led to even more excitement around the increasingly popular gamma camera, as there was now easy access to a radioisotope which was perfect for use with the gamma camera, as ^{99m}Tc is a relatively low energy radionuclide with ideal nuclear properties for gamma imaging [12]. This ease of access led to the development of many new radiotracers for other medical applications using ^{99m}Tc as the radioactive source, and a swift decline in the price tag of the table top generator.

NaF, on the other hand, is produced by a particle accelerator or cyclotron [13], and in the 1960s, cyclotrons were not as abundant as they are today. Also, with the less optimal nuclear properties of NaF, for example, a relatively short half-life, it is necessary to have access to a reasonably closely located cyclotron in order to obtain enough radionuclide for use [13–16].

Yet another blow to NaF was the discovery of ^{99m}Tc-methyl diphosphonate (^{99m}Tc-MDP) in 1971 by McAfee and Subramanian, which is a bone seeking agent using the easily accessible ^{99m}Tc radionuclide combined with a relatively simply, and cost effectively, made compound, which is still routinely used in nuclear medicine for evaluation of many diseases of the bones [17]. The abandonment of NaF was not based on limitations of the tracer itself, but rather due to high cost and the now widely available ^{99m}Tc-MDP. Again, we have come a long way since the 1970s. Enter: The Positron Emission Tomography (PET) scanner.

The first PET scanner was built in 1961 at Brookhaven National Laboratory and is based on the idea of detecting two gamma photons traveling in opposite directions, produced where uptake of the radiotracer occurs [18]. This scanner is called a positron scanner because it detects radiotracers which emit photons produced by the interaction of a positron with an electron, also known as an annihilation event [18].

The PET scanner gained significant popularity following experiments using [^{18}F] fluoro-deoxy glucose (FDG), which is the glucose analog used to detect areas of varying metabolic activity, which is of particular importance in consideration of the Warburg Effect and its relation to actively dividing cancer cells [19–21].

The first dose of FDG for human use was prepared in August 1976 at Brookhaven Laboratory, and flown from Long Island to Philadelphia where Dr. Abass Alavi at the University of Pennsylvania was the first person to inject this radiotracer into humans. Following injection, he imaged the brain of a volunteer medical student [20–22]. Then, they proceeded to image the entirety of the body, and from that point on, imaging of physiology in Nuclear Medicine would never be the same [22].

In 1998 following development of the hybrid PET/CT scanner, as well as the appearance of more medical cyclotrons for production of 18F, widespread use of PET/CT imaging transpired [23, 24].

PET/CT is currently standard of care in many malignant diseases and therefore found in many communities. Cyclotron sites have also popped up nationwide and can provide large geographic areas with positron emitting agents, such as 18F, and thus, NaF.

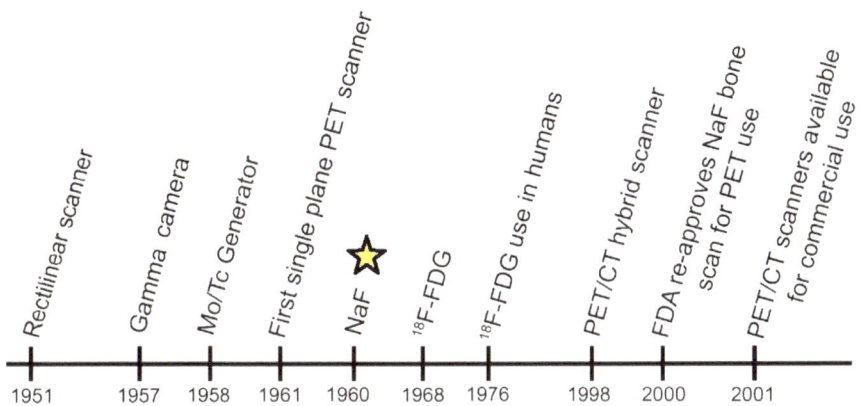

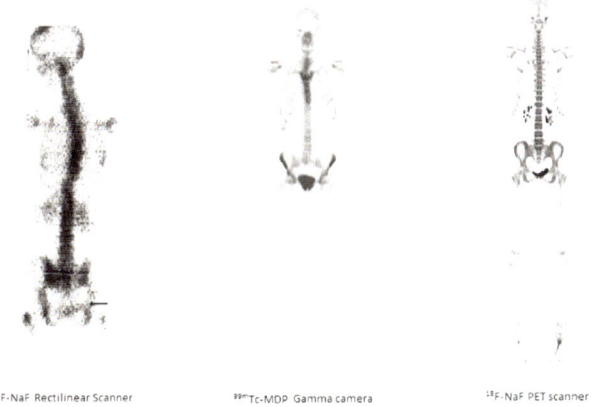

18F-NaF Rectilinear Scanner   99mTc-MDP Gamma camera   18F-NaF PET scanner

The availability of PET/CT scanners and more readily available positron production have led to the resurgence of interest in NaF use as a scanning agent.

More recently, the ability of NaF to identify atherosclerotic plaque diseases has led to the identification of new tricks, for this old dog [25, 26, 29].

1.2   Radiotracer Properties and Technique

NaF is a cyclotron produced positron agent, which has a half-life of 110 min, and emits photons with energies of 511 keV, visualized by positron emission tomography [9, 16].

NaF is used for the assessment of bone metabolism, primarily in the evaluation of malignancy and metastatic disease of the bony skeleton. $Na^{18}F$ uptake is a reflection of both blood flow to the bones and bone remodeling [28].

The radiotracer is injected intravenously and once diffused through capillaries feeding the bones where turnover is highest, the ^{18}F is exchanged for a hydroxyl group in the bone mineral hydroxyapatite, leading to the formation of ^{18}F-fluorapatite (Fig. 1.1).

Fig. 1.1 Incorporation of ^{18}F from NaF into the hydroxyapatite crystals of the mineral bone matrix to form the radioactive fluorapatite crystals (illustration by Kelley Kage)

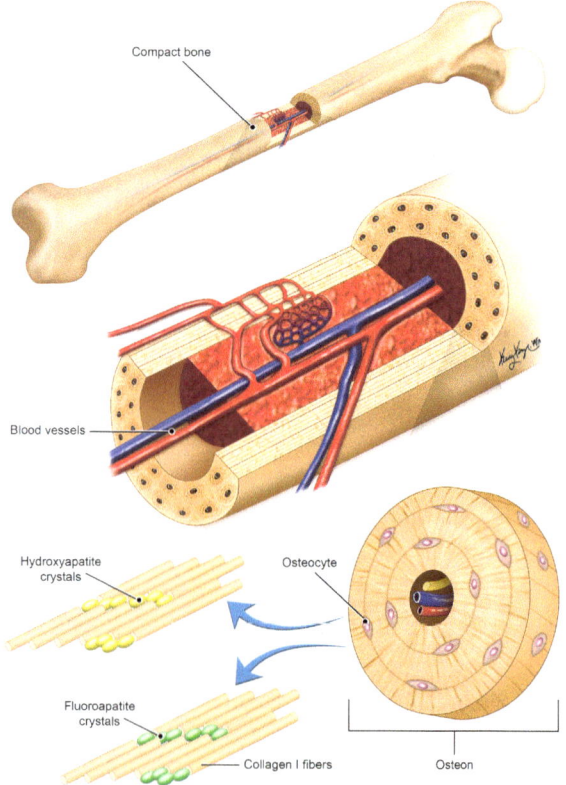

^{18}F adheres to bone via absorption and is incorporated into bone at twice the rate as of phosphonates, such as ^{99m}Tc-MDP [30]. Unlike other bone imaging phosphonates, ^{18}F does not bind to serum protein. However, 30% of ^{99m}Tc-MDP immediately binds to protein following injection, and 70% at 24 h post injection [3, 27].

NaF demonstrates rapid clearance with approximately 10% remaining in the blood after 1 h, with the bone, bone marrow, and urinary bladder serving as the target and critical organs [27].

1.3   Patient Preparation

Na^{18}F requires little to no patient preparation including no dietary or activity restrictions, and no discontinuation of any medications. It is important, however, that the patient is well hydrated before and after imaging.

Patients are required to lie in a supine and stationary position for approximately 30 min to 1 h, depending on the type of scan necessary to address the clinical question. Patients are encouraged to take any prescribed anxiolytics and/or pain medications prior to imaging in order to comply with these requirements.

In order to maintain low radiation exposure to the general public, family members are not allowed to remain with patients, and patients are kept in a confined safety area of the clinic during and after radiotracer injection, until the scan is complete. Patients who are currently breastfeeding are instructed to pump enough milk for 24 h prior to scanning, or use formulated supplement for 24 h, to allow for proper time for the radiotracer to leave the body.

Special circumstances, such as patients under the age of 18, or those with reduced mental capacity, may have a family member or caretaker present as long as they are properly educated on radiation safety. Female family members who are pregnant may not be allowed to accompany such patients.

There are no medical contraindications to Na^{18}F scanning. However, certain patient-specific conditions and staff radiation exposures may restrict the ability to scan; for example, pregnancy, body weight greater than 181.4 kg, patients who have received high density contrast within 72 h, critically ill patients, and patients requiring general anesthesia.

1.4   Technique

The Na^{18}F radiotracer dose in adults is typically between 185 and 370 MBq (5–10 mCi), using higher doses for larger patients.

In pediatric patients dosing is weight based using a standard of 2.22 MBq/kg (0.06 mCi/kg), and a range with a minimum dose of 18.5 MBq and a maximum dose of 185 MBq (0.5–5 mCi).

The radiotracer is administered intravenously, although oral administration has been performed in the past, and due to rapid intestinal absorption, this method of administration may be used as an alternative to those without venous access; however, this technique has not been adequately vetted [3, 31, 32].

Following injection the patient is held in a localization room for approximately 45–60 min in order for adequate distribution throughout the body. Following emptying of the bladder, the patient is placed supine, onto the PET/CT scanner and imaged from the vertex of the skull to the toes, or based on the patient specific parameters requested by the ordering physician [31, 32].

Acknowledgment I would like to thank Richelle D. Millican, Positron Emission Tomography Manager at MD Anderson Cancer Center, for her expert contribution to the PET imaging protocol section of this chapter.

References

1. Rontgen WK. Ueber eine neue Art von Strahlen (on a new kind of rays). Sitzungsberichte der Würzburger Physik-medic. Gesellschaft. 1895 [translation from Nature 53: 274–276, 1896].
2. Thomas AMK, Banerjee AK. The history of radiology. Cary: Oxford University Press; 2013.
3. Blau M, Nagler W, Bender M. Fluorine-18: a new isotope for bone scanning. J Nucl Med. 1962;3:332–4.
4. Cassen B, Curtis L, Reed C, Libby R. Instrumentation for ^{131}I use in medical studies. Nucleonics. 1951;9:46–50.
5. Williams LE. Anniversary paper: nuclear medicine: fifty years and still counting. Med Phys. 2008;35(7):3020–9. https://doi.org/10.1118/1.2936217.
6. Anger HO. Use of a gamma-ray pinhole camera for in vivo studies. Nature. 1952;170: 200–1.
7. Fowler JS, Wolf AP. The synthesis of carbon-11, fluorine-18 and nitrogen-13 labeled radiotracers for biomedical applications, National Academy of Sciences—National Research Council. Nuclear Science Series: Monographs. Upton: Brookhaven National Lab; 1982.
8. Yano Y, Van Dyke DC, Verdon TA Jr, Anger HO. Cyclotron-produced 157Dy compared with ^{18}F for bone scanning using the whole-body scanner and scintillation camera. J Nucl Med. 1971 Dec;12(12):815–21.
9. Powsner ER, Palmer MR, Powsner RA. Essentials of nuclear medicine physics and instrumentation. 3rd ed. Hoboken: Wiley; 2013.
10. Tucker WD, Greene MW, Weis AJ, Murrenhoff A. Methods of preparation of some carrier-free radioisotopes involving sorption on alumina. Upton: Brookhaven National Lab; 1958.
11. Stang LG Jr, Tucker WD, Doering RF, Weiss AJ, Greene MW, Banks HO Jr. Development of methods for the production of certain short-lived radioisotopes. Int J Appl Radiat Isot. 1957;2:252. https://doi.org/10.1016/0020-708X(57)90233-8.
12. Harper PV, Lathrop KA, Jiminez F, Fink R, Gottschalk A. Technetium—99m as a scanning agent. Radiology. 1965;85:101.
13. Clark JC, Silvesterj DJ. A cyclotron method for the production of Fluorine-18. Int J Appl Radiat. 1966;17:151.
14. Carlson CH, Armstrong WD, Singer L. Distribution, migration and binding of whole blood fluoride evaluated with radiofluoride. Am J Phys. 1960;199:187–9.
15. Weber DA, Greenberg EJ, Dimich A, et al. Kinetics of radionuclides used for bone studies. J Nucl Med. 1969;10:8–17.

16. Hawkins RA, Choi Y, Huang SC, et al. Evaluation of the skeletal kinetics of fluorine-18-fluoride ion with PET. J Nucl Med. 1992;33:633–42.
17. Subramanian G, McAfee J. A new complex of ⁹⁹ᵐTc for skeletal imaging. Radiology. 1971;99:192–6.
18. Phelps ME, Hoffman EJ, Mullani NA, Ter-Pogossian MM. Application of annihilation coincidence detection to transaxial reconstruction tomography. J Nucl Med. 1975;16:210–24.
19. Pacák J, Točík Z, Černý M. Synthesis of 2-deoxy-2-fluoro-D-glucose. J Chem Soc D. 1969;2:77.
20. Ido T, Wan CN, Casella V, Fowler JS, Wolf AP, Reivich M, Kuhl DE. Labeled 2-deoxy-D-glucose analogs. ¹⁸F-labeled 2-deoxy-2-fluoro-D-glucose, 2-deoxy-2-fluoro-D-mannose and 14C-2-deoxy-2-fluoro-D-glucose. J Labelled Compd Radiopharm. 1978;24:174–83.
21. Gogvadze V, Zhivotovsky B, Orrenius S. The Warburg effect and mitochondrial stability in cancer cells. Mol Aspects Med. 2010;31(1):60–74.
22. Mohammadi H. Professor Abass Alavi, distinguished medical scientist. Arch Iran Med. 2015;18:458–60.
23. Townsend DW, Wensveen M, Byars LG. A rotating PET scanner using BGO block detectors: design, performance and applications. J Nucl Med. 1993;34:1367–76.
24. Beyer T, Townsend DW, Brun T. A combined PET/CT scanner for clinical oncology. J Nucl Med. 2000;41:1369–79.
25. Joshi NV, Vesey A, Williams MC, Shah AS, Newby DE, et al. ¹⁸F-fluoride positron emission tomography for identification of ruptured and high-risk coronary atherosclerotic plaques: a prospective clinical trial. Lancet. 2014;383(9918):705–13.
26. Forsythe RO, Dweck MR, McBride OMB, et al. ¹⁸F–sodium fluoride uptake in abdominal aortic aneurysms: the SoFIA3 study. J Am Coll Cardiol. 2018;71(5):513–23.
27. Czernin J, Satyamurthy N, Schiepers C. Molecular mechanisms of bone ¹⁸F-NaF deposition. J Nucl Med. 2010;51(12):1826–9.
28. Fogelman I, Cook G, Israel O, Van der Wall H. Positron emission tomography and bone metastases. Semin Nucl Med. 2005;35:135–42.
29. Ordonez AA, DeMarco VP, Klunk MH, Pokkali S, Jain SK. Imaging chronic tuberculous lesions using sodium (¹⁸F) fluoride positron emission tomography in mice. Mol Imaging Biol. 2015;17(5):609–14.
30. Iagaru AH, Mittra E, Colletti PM, Jadvar H. Bone-targeted imaging and radionuclide therapy in prostate Cancer. J Nucl Med. 2016;57(Suppl 3):19S–24S.
31. Segall G, Delbeke D, Stabin MG, Even-Sapir E, Fair J, Sajdak R, Smith GT. SNM practice guideline for sodium ¹⁸F-fluoride PET/CT bone scans 1.0. J Nucl Med. 2010;51(11):1813–20.
32. Beheshti M, Mottaghy FM, Paycha F, Behrendt FFF, Van den Wyngaert T, Fogelman I, Strobel K, Celli M, Fanti S, Giammarile F, Krause B, Langsteger W. ¹⁸F-NaF PET/CT: EANM procedure guidelines for bone imaging. Eur J Nucl Med Mol Imaging. 2015;42:1767.

^{18}F-Fluoride Imaging: Normal Variants and Artifacts

2

Guofan Xu

Contents

Sodium fluoride labeled with fluorine 18 (sodium fluoride F18 [^{18}F-NaF]) is a bone seeking positron-emitting radiopharmaceutical tracer. ^{18}F-NaF PET/CT provides great sensitivity and specificity in the detection of bone metastases. Uptake of ^{18}F sodium fluoride reflects blood flow and bony remodeling. When combining with the CT component of the PET/CT, it allows better morphologic characterization of the functional findings and achieves more accurate differentiation with improved specificity.

In this chapter, a review of the indications, normal imaging appearances, and artifacts of ^{18}F-NaF PET/CT in the evaluation of skeletal disease are provided, with an emphasis on oncologic imaging.

The original version of this chapter was revised. The correction to this chapter can be found at https://doi.org/10.1007/978-3-030-23577-2_12

G. Xu (✉)
Department of Nuclear Medicine, University of Texas MD Anderson Cancer Center, Houston, TX, USA
e-mail: GXu2@mdanderson.org

© Springer Nature Switzerland AG 2020
K. Kairemo, H. A. Macapinlac (eds.), *Sodium Fluoride PET/CT in Clinical Use*, Clinicians' Guides to Radionuclide Hybrid Imaging, https://doi.org/10.1007/978-3-030-23577-2_2

9

2.1   Introduction

The axial skeleton consists of 80 bones:

- 29 bones in the head—(8 cranial and 14 facial bones) and then also 7 associated bones (6 auditory ossicles and the Hyoid Bone)
- 25 bones of the thorax (the sternum and 24 ribs)
- 26 bones in the vertebral column (24 vertebrae, the sacrum, and the coccyx)

  The appendicular skeleton consists of 134 bones:

- 4 bones in the shoulder girdle (clavicle and scapula each side)
- 6 bones in the arm and forearm (humerus, ulna, and radius)
- 58 bones in the hands (carpals 16, metacarpals 10, phalanges 28, and sesamoid 4)
- 2 pelvic bones
- 8 bones in the legs (femur, tibia, patella, and fibula)
- 56 bones in the feet (tarsals, metatarsals, phalanges, and sesamoid)

2.2   Normal NaF Image

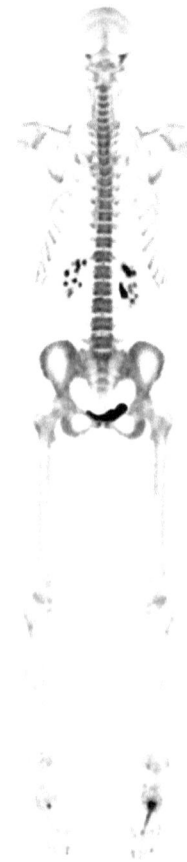

Normal physiologic biodistribution of F-18-NaF in a healthy 23-year-old woman. Anterior and lateral maximum intensity projection (MIP) images show normal pattern of radiotracer uptake within the skeleton. There is also prominent radiotracer uptake in the kidneys and the bladder from excreted urine. Of note, there is increased radiotracer uptake in the metatarsal bones of bilateral feet, which is commonly seen in the patients and likely due to stress-related bone remodeling.

Uptake of ^{18}F-NaF is not tumor specific, and nonmalignant processes can show avid radiotracer uptake, including normal growth plate, arthritis, trauma, and benign osseous processes such as fibrous dysplasia and Paget disease. The degree of radiotracer uptake cannot be used to differentiate benign from malignant lesions [1].

Normal growth plates in pediatric population

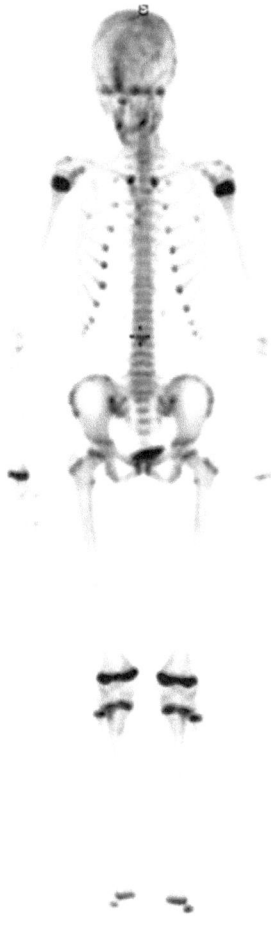

^{18}F-NaF PET/CT images in a 17-year-old female. MIP image shows physiologic uptake in the skeleton and growth plates with normal prominence of costochondral junctions. With permission from Dr. Ismet Sarikaya [2].

2.3   Bone Marrow Expansion

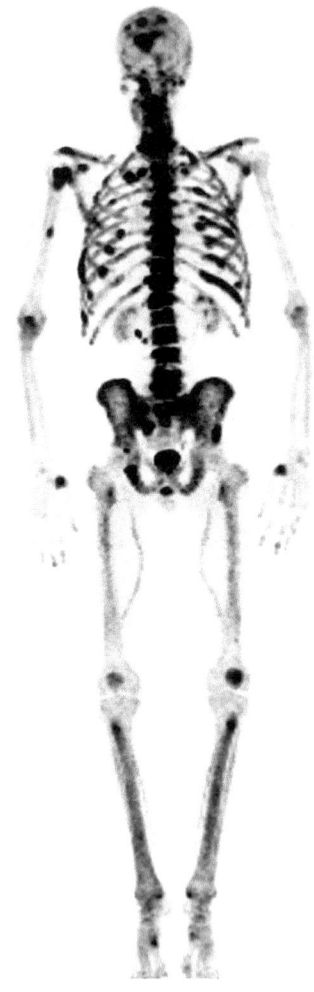

[18]F-NaF PET/CT whole-body MIP image shows diffusely increased radio-tracer uptake in the distal bilateral legs, which indicates bone marrow expansion.

2.4   Artifact Related to Arm Down Position

Placing the arms down during the acquisition, particularly in a large-sized patient, can create photopenic or cold areas in the bone and soft tissues. These cold areas are usually not seen on the non-attenuation corrected images.

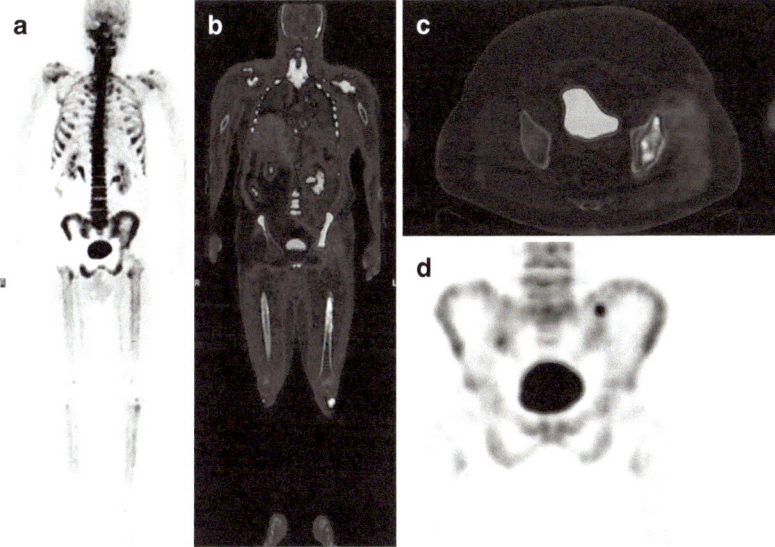

^{18}F-NaF PET/CT images of a patient in the arms-down position. MIP image (a), and coronal and transaxial PET/CT fusion images (b, c) show a photopenic area mainly in the right hip and the surrounding soft tissues. Repeat PET/CT imaging in the hip region in the arms-up position shows normal uptake in the bones (d). With permission from Dr. Ismet Sarikaya [2].

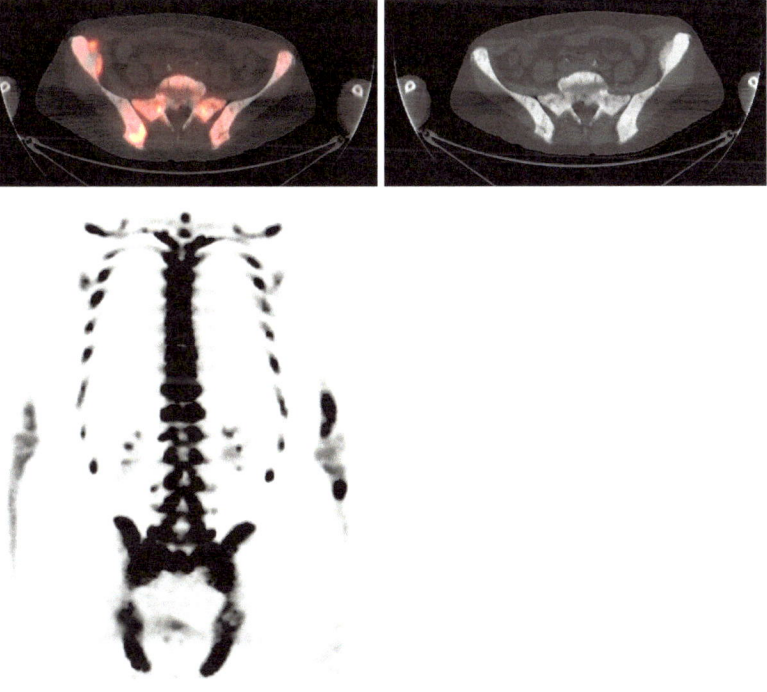

2.5 Motion Artifacts

The total scan time for ^{18}F NaF PET/CT is shorter than ^{99m}Tc-MDP whole body bone scan, which could decrease the potentials for motion artifacts from the patients. The possible motion-related artifacts are shown in the below images.

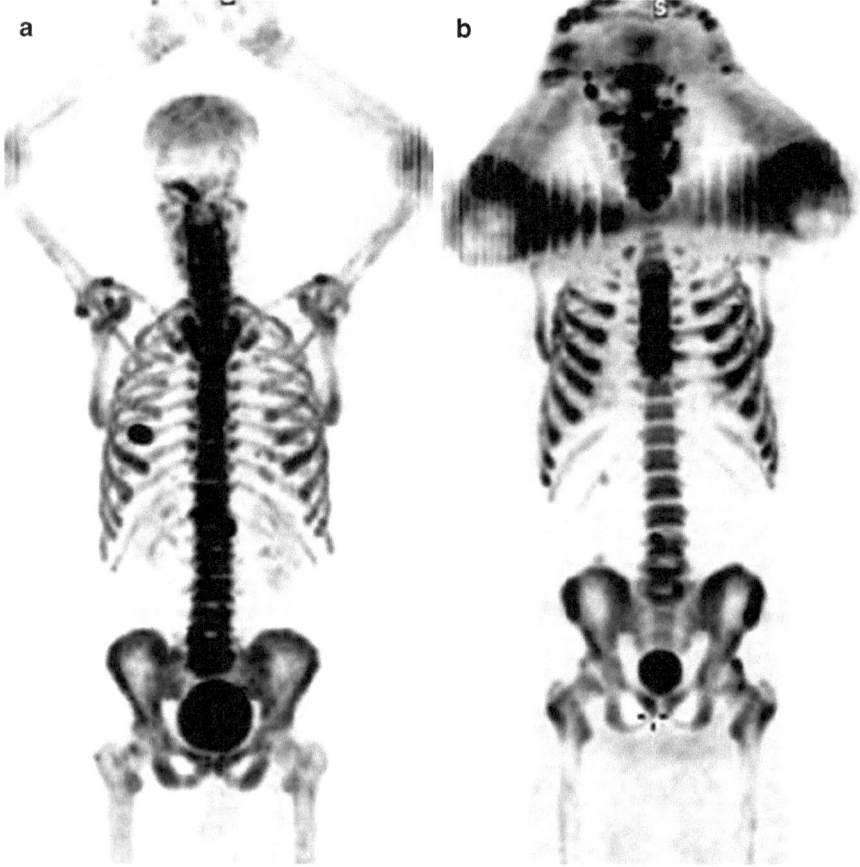

MIP (maximum intensity projection) images of two patients showing a horizontal linear area of reduced uptake in the head (a) and streak artifacts around elbows (b). With permission from Dr. Ismet Sarikaya [2].

2.6   Misregistration Artifact

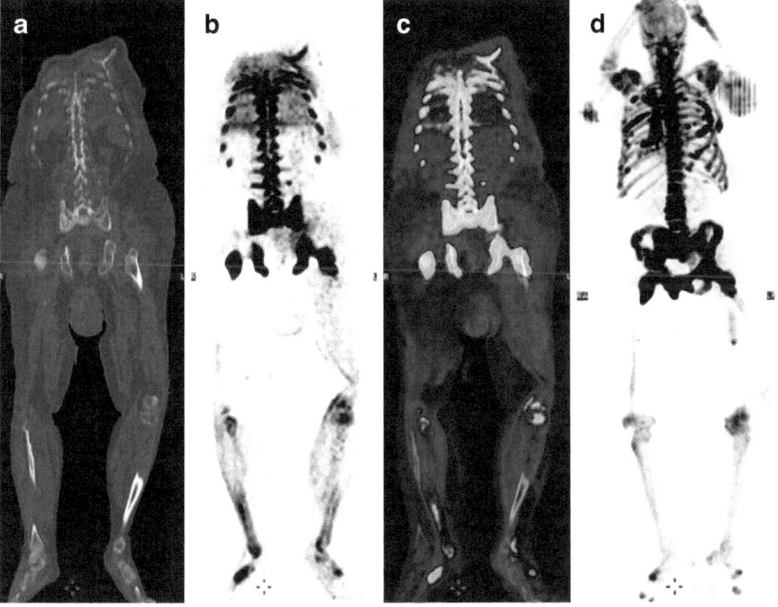

There is significant misregistration artifacts in both legs (b–d) because of patient motion. Non-AC PET images could help to detect CT overcorrection artifacts. If there is motion during PET acquisition, repeat images should be obtained [3]. With permission from Dr. Ismet Sarikaya [2].

2.7   Orthopedic Hardware-Related Artifact

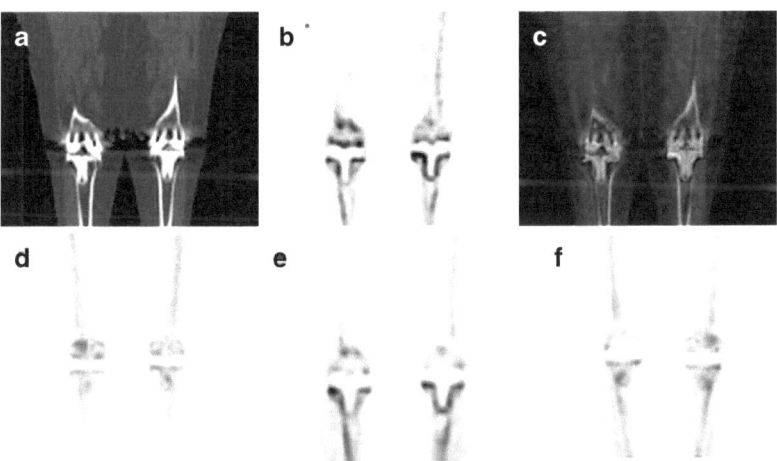

Coronal CT, PET, PET/CT fusion, and MIP images of the knees (a–d) show orthopedic hardware in both the knees with surrounding increased activity. Coronal non-
AC PET and non-AC MIP images (e, f) show less intense uptake around orthopedic
hardwares in the knees. With permission from Dr. Ismet Sarikaya [2].

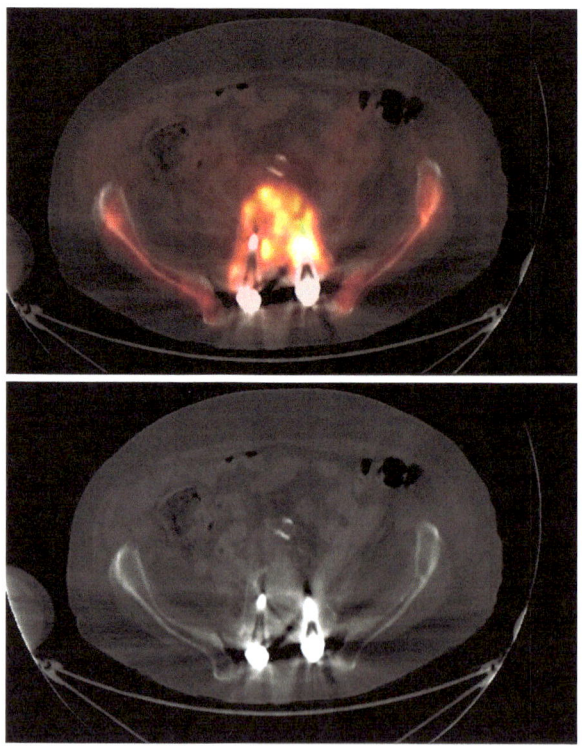

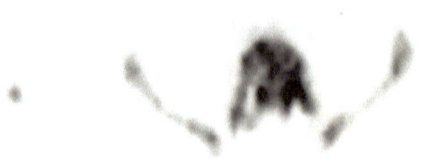

Axial PET/CT fusion, CT, and PET images of the pelvis show spinal fusion
hardware in the L5 vertebral body with surrounding increased activity. The prostheses are photopenic on PET.

References

1. Bastawrous S, et al. Newer PET application with an old tracer: role of ^{18}F-NaF skeletal PET/CT in oncologic practice. RadioGraphics. 2014;34:1295–316.
2. Sarikaya I, et al. Normal bone and soft tissue distribution of fluorine-18 sodium fluoride and artifacts on ^{18}F NaF PET/CT bone scan: a pictorial review. Nucl Med Commun. 2017;38:810–9.
3. Simpson CD, et al. FDG PET/CT: artifacts and pitfalls. Contemp Diagn Radiol. 2017;40(5):1.

Sodium Fluoride Imaging in Oncology

3

Kalevi Kairemo and Homer A. Macapinlac

Contents

3.1 Introduction

[18]F-NaF PET/CT has established its place in the oncologic clinical routine. It has essential role in initial staging, detection of suspected first osseous metastasis, suspected progression of osseous metastasis, or treatment monitoring in many types of cancer, such as prostate, lung, and breast cancer.

K. Kairemo (✉)
Department of Nuclear Medicine and Molecular Radiotherapy, Docrates Cancer Center, Helsinki, Finland

Department of Nuclear Medicine, University of Texas MD Anderson Cancer Center, Houston, TX, USA

H. A. Macapinlac
Department of Nuclear Medicine, University of Texas MD Anderson Cancer Center, Houston, TX, USA

© Springer Nature Switzerland AG 2020
K. Kairemo, H. A. Macapinlac (eds.), *Sodium Fluoride PET/CT in Clinical Use*, Clinicians' Guides to Radionuclide Hybrid Imaging, https://doi.org/10.1007/978-3-030-23577-2_3

The Society for Nuclear Medicine has published guidelines for ^{18}F-NaF PET/CT [1]. Bone uptake of ^{18}F-NaF reflects bone remodeling, and the uptake of ^{18}F-NaF is part of the mineralization of bone matrix. ^{18}F- is exchanged for OH$^-$ so hydroxyapatite bone matrix is transformed into fluoroapatite, indicating that high uptake of ^{18}F-NaF reflects bone reactions to bone metastases, not to cancer itself. Therefore, positive findings with ^{18}F-NaF PET/CT may be due to both benign and malignant bone disorders. In spite of this, the US National Oncologic PET Registry (NOPR) has collected NaF PET results linked to Medicare claims by imaging initial staging, detection of new suspected skeletal metastases, suspected progression of skeletal disease, or assessing treatment response in prostate, lung, or breast cancer. In an analysis from this NOPR registry of 21,167 ^{18}F-NaF PET/CT studies, the results were associated with subsequent hospice claims and with patient survival. ^{18}F-NaF-PET provides important information on the presence of osseous metastasis and prognosis to assist patients and their physicians when making decisions on whether to select palliative care and transition to hospice or whether to continue treatment [2].

In this chapter the use of ^{18}F-NaF PET/CT in prostate, breast, lung, thyroid, and renal cell cancer will be reviewed.

3.2 Prostate Cancer

Some international recommendations already include ^{18}F-NaF as a radiotracer for skeletal imaging [3]. PET/CT technology has exhibited higher spatial resolution and substantially greater sensitivity than conventional gamma cameras, resulting in higher image quality for a skeletal PET than for planar bone scintigraphy or SPECT [4–6].

^{18}F-NaF has been used initial staging, detection of new suspected skeletal metastases, suspected progression of skeletal disease, or assessing treatment response in prostate. Chapter 6 describes in a more detailed manner the methods for response criteria.

The ^{18}F-NaF fluoride PET/CT methodology allows for the simultaneous characterization of the alterations of metastatic bone density and the tracer uptake, which both are well-established markers of lesion severity and may be essential in judging the necessity of early implementation of radionuclide therapies for bony pain palliation and treatment. For instance, most lytic lesions are not detectable at bone scintigraphy. It has been reported that in cancer patients with multiple skeletal metastases an increased ^{18}F-NaF-fluoride uptake is detected both in lesions with sclerotic characteristics on CT and in mixed sclerotic and lytic metastases [7].

There is a small meta-analysis about ^{18}F-NaF PET/CT scans: of 3918 patients, 1289 (33%) had positive scans [8]. In the NOPR [9], the indication for the PET/CT was reflected in the PET/CT findings: 14% of patients had a positive ^{18}F-NaF PET/CT at staging; 29% of the patients had positive ^{18}F-NaF PET/CT if the examination was an initial test for bone metastases; 76% of the patients had positive ^{18}F-NaF PET/CT if the examination was requested as a test for progressive bone metastases.

^{18}F-NaF and ^{18}F-Choline PET/CT had similar diagnostic accuracy at staging for patients with prostate cancer but ^{18}F-Choline has higher specificity at restaging for recurrence [10]. Patients with positive ^{18}F-NaF PET/CT scans have a high risk of having dissemination of prostate cancer to the bones.

Bone metastases occur in nearly all patients with castration resistant prostate cancer and are the primary cause of disability, impaired quality of life, and death, due to an increased risk of pathologic fractures, spinal cord or nerve root compression, and hypercalcemia of malignancy [11]. In this context, the skeletal involvement from prostate cancer can be assessed using ^{18}F-NaF-fluoride PET/CT. This imaging modality allows the identification and quantification of bone metastatic lesions [12, 13].

Current drugs for the treatment of bone metastases also include ADT and systemic chemotherapy but monoclonal antibodies, analgesics, EBRT, radiopharmaceuticals, and bisphosphonates, specifically target osseous disease alone or in combination. However, ^{18}F-NaF-fluoride PET/CT is best in the evaluation of bone targeted therapies and in bone dominant metastatic prostate cancer.

This ^{18}F-fluoride PET/CT methodology can be used for assessing the final outcome of many treatments [6]. The Na^{18}F burden data is convincing (Chap. 5), because serum markers, such as alkaline phosphatase (AFOS) or prostate-specific antigen (PSA), seldom reflect small changes in the overall cancer burden. Figure 3.1 demonstrates

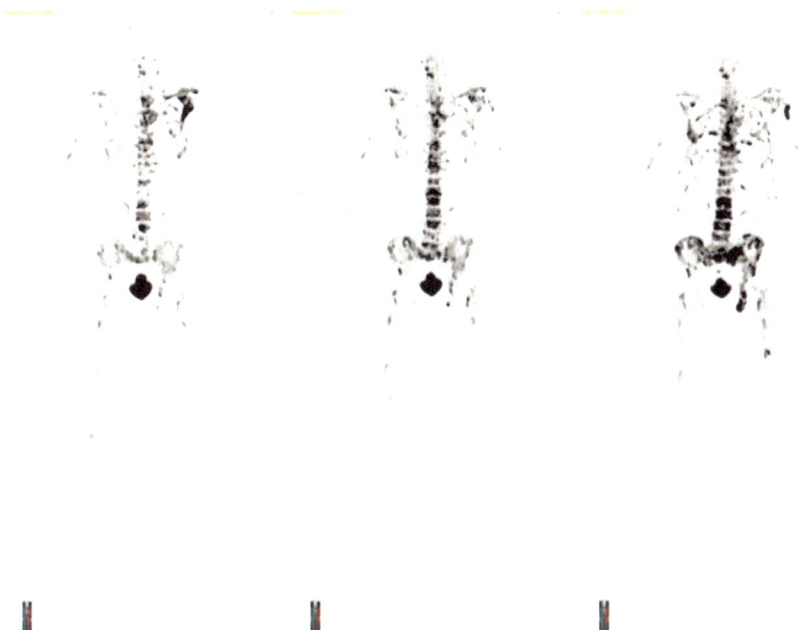

Fig. 3.1 ^{18}F-fluoride PET/CT changes in skeletal metastases at baseline, after 3 cycles, and after 6 cycles of ^{223}Ra-treatment for pain palliation from skeletal disease. Reprinted with permission of Bentham Science Publishers from Kairemo et al. [6]

[18]F-fluoride PET/CT changes in skeletal metastases at baseline, after 3 cycles and after 6 cycles of [223]Ra-treatment for pain palliation from skeletal disease.

3.3 Breast Cancer

Osseous metastases in breast cancer are in approximately 50% osteoblastic, whereas in prostate cancer osteoblastic metastases occur in more than 80% of metastases based on histomorphometry [14].

The largest study in the literature about NaF PET/CT in osseous metastases in breast cancer consisted of 118 patients [15]. In this Dutch study F-NaF PET/CT detected bone metastases in 42% with an accuracy of 0.93. The scan results led to a change in patient management in 25%. In the evaluation of bone pain, an explanation for pain was found in 71% of the scans, benign pathology in 66%, and bone metastases in 5%. Indications for ^{18}F-NaF PET/CT included primary staging (12%), follow-up (31%), bone pain (52%), abnormal laboratory findings (5%), and evaluation of equivocal osseous lesions on other imaging modalities (3%). Bone metastases were found in 42%, whereas 53% of the scans were negative and 5% yielded equivocal results. Correlation with the reference standard yielded a sensitivity of 0.96, a specificity of 0.91, a positive predictive value of 0.89, a negative predictive value of 0.97, and an accuracy of 0.93 [15].

In another study from Brazil [16], the skeletal tumor burden (TLF_{10}) on ^{18}F-Fluoride PET/CT images of 107 female breast cancer patients was quantified, 40 for primary staging and the remainder for restaging after therapy. Bone metastases were present in 49 patients, and the median follow-up time was 19.5 months. On multivariable analysis, skeletal tumor burden was significantly and independently associated with overall survival ($p < 0.0001$) and progression free-survival ($p < 0.0001$). The simple presence of bone metastases was associated with time to bone event ($p = 0.045$) [16].

There has been some attempts to characterize the ^{18}F-NaF behavior skeletal metastases of breast cancer in more detailed manner, especially in relation to prognosis and endocrine treatment, but results are very preliminary. ^{18}F-fluoride metabolic flux to bone mineral (Ki) by positron emission tomography/computed tomography (PET/CT) may provide incremental value in response assessment of bone metastases in breast cancer, because a significant mean percentage increase in Ki from baseline occurred in the 4 patients with clinical progressive disease compared with SUV_{max} (89.7% vs 41.9; $p < 0.001$) [17]. After 8 weeks of endocrine treatment for bone-predominant metastatic breast cancer, Ki more reliably differentiated disease progression from non-progression: In the 4 patients with clinical progressive disease, mean Ki significantly increased (>25%) in all, whereas in the 8 non-progrediating patients, Ki decreased or remained stable in 7 [17].

Additionally, a prospective study has been performed to test ^{18}F-FDG PET and ^{18}F-NaF PET to predict time to skeletal related events (tSRE) and time-to-progression

(TTP), and overall survival (OS) in patients with bone-dominant metastatic breast cancer [18]. 28 patients with were imaged with ^{18}F-FDG PET and ^{18}F-NaF PET prior to new therapy and again approximately 4 months later. Changes in ^{18}F-FDG PET parameters during therapy were predictive of tSRE and TTP, but not OS. Serial ^{18}F-NaF PET was associated with OS, because an increase in the uptake between scans of up to 5 lesions by ^{18}F-NaF PET was associated with longer OS ($P = 0.027$). NaF was not useful for predicting TTP or tSRE in these patients [18].

3.4 Lung Cancer

The only large study in the literature compared the diagnostic accuracy of F-labeled sodium fluoride (^{18}F-NaF) PET/CT with 99m-technetium methylene diphosphonate (Tc-MDP) single photon emission computed tomography (SPECT) to detect bone metastases (BMs) in patients with preoperative lung cancer. Patients with lung cancer ($n = 181$) were examined with ^{18}F-NaF PET/CT, and another 167 patients with lung cancer were examined with Tc-MDP SPECT [20]. Sensitivity and specificity of PET/CT were significantly better than that of SPECT when equivocal reading was categorized as malignant or benign ($P < 0.05$). Based on lesions-based analysis, SPECT produced 26 equivocal lesions of 333 lesions, but PET/CT produced only 5 equivocal lesions of 991 lesions. PET/CT was significantly better than SPECT in the aspect of producing equivocal patients ($\chi = 58.141$, $P < 0.001$). Sensitivity and specificity of PET/CT were significantly better than that of SPECT when equivocal reading was categorized as malignant or benign ($P < 0.05$). ^{18}F-NaF PET/CT is a highly sensitive and specific modality for the detection of BMs in patients with preoperative lung cancer. It is better than conventional Tc-MDP SPECT in detecting BMs in patients with preoperative lung cancer [19].

3.5 Thyroid Cancer

Two small studies have compared diagnostic performance of ^{18}F-NaF PET/CT with bone scintigraphy of the detection of thyroid cancer bone metastases. In a Korean study of the 17 suspected bone lesions in six (papillary:follicular = 2:4) patients, 10 were metastatic and 7 benign [20]. Compared to BS, bone PET/CT exhibited superior sensitivity (10/10 = 100% vs. 2/10 = 20%, $p = 0.008$) and accuracy (14/17 = 82.4% vs. 7/17 = 41.2%, $p < 0.025$). The specificity (4/7 = 57.1%) of bone PET/CT was not significantly different from that of BS (5/7 = 71.4%, $p > 0.05$) [20].

A Japanese study consisted of 11 patients who had been suspected of having bone metastases after total thyroidectomy and were hospitalized to be given ^{131}I therapy [21]. Metastases were confirmed in 24 (13.6%) of 176 bone segments in

9 of the 11 patients. The sensitivity of ^{18}F-fluoridePET/CT was significantly higher than those of ^{18}F-FDG PET/CT and [99]mTc bone scintigraphy (planar) ($p < 0.05$) [21].

The original study of 35 patients with known or suspected bone metastases from thyroid (papillary:follicular = 9:26) carcinoma evaluated the anatomical distribution and metabolic behavior of bone metastases using bone scintigraphy, whole-body iodine scintigraphy, F-18-Na-F PET, and CT or MRI [22]. The anatomical distribution of 43 bone metastases found in 18 patients was as follows: spine, 42%; skull, 2%; thorax, 16%; femur, 9%; pelvis, 26%; humerus and clavicle, 5%. All metastases were osteolytic on x-ray and two-thirds (29/43) presented a missing or very limited osteosclerotic bone reaction on F-18 PET. The combination bone scintigraphy and whole-body iodine scintigraphy revealed all the metastases, but neither of them alone. The findings, including a low sensitivity of NaF (33%), are explained by missing or only weak osteosclerotic bone reaction in thyroid cancer bone metastases [22].

3.6   Renal Cell Cancer

Two studies have compared diagnostic performance of ^{18}F-NaF PET/CT with bone scintigraphy or the detection of renal cell cancer (RCC) bone metastases. ^{18}F-NaF PET/CT is significantly more sensitive at detecting RCC skeletal metastases than conventional bone scintigraphy or CT. Seventy-seven lesions in ten patients were diagnosed as malignant: 100% were identified by ^{18}F-NaF PET/CT, 46% by CT, and 29% by bone scintigraphy/SPECT [23]. Standard-of-care imaging with CT and bone scintigraphy identified 65% of the metastases reported by ^{18}F-NaF PET/CT. On an individual patient basis, ^{18}F-NaF PET/CT detected more RCC metastases than (99m)Tc-MDP bone scintigraphy/SPECT or CT alone ($P = 0.007$). The SUV mean and SUV max of the malignant lesions were significantly greater than those of the benign lesions ($P < 0.001$) [23]. The detection of occult bone metastases could greatly alter patient management, particularly in the context when standard-of-care imaging is negative for skeletal metastases.

Another study reports similar results: Overall, F-fluoride PET/CT showed a sensitivity of 100%, specificity of 94.4%, positive predictive value of 94.7%, negative predictive value of 100%, and accuracy of 97.2% [24]. It demonstrated a total of 134 skeletal lesions, of which 101 were characterized as metastasis and 33 as benign. Corresponding CT changes were seen for 129/134 lesions. The mean SUVmax of the lesions was 30 ± 48. F-Fluoride PET/CT and F-FDG PET/CT showed similar accuracy for visualization of bone metastasis (93.7 vs. 100%; $P - 0.993$). However, F-FDG PET/CT additionally demonstrated extraskeletal metastasis in 6/16 patients. No significant difference was seen between the accuracies of BS and F-fluoride PET/CT for visualization of bone metastasis (93.7 vs. 100%; $P = 0.115$), but the former showed significantly more skeletal lesions (91 vs. 44; $P < 0.0001$). In 4/22 patients (18%) with negative BS, F-fluoride PET/CT demonstrated skeletal metastases [24].

3.7 Medullary Thyroid Carcinoma (MTC)

Medullary thyroid carcinoma (MTC) is a rare condition, and a few cases have been reported in the literature where ^{18}F-NaF PET/CT has been useful in the differential diagnosis of MTC. ^{18}F-NaF PET/CT could be helpful not only to the detection of bone metastases but also to the detection of calcified soft tissue metastases in patients with MTC, such as pulmonary and lymph node metastases [25], brain [26], and liver metastases [27]. Then this finding can be used in planning and selection of the therapy [28].

References

1. Segall G, Delbeke D, Stabin MG, et al. SNM practice guideline for sodium ^{18}F-fluoride PET/CT bone scans 1.0. J Nucl Med. 2010;51:1813–20.
2. Gareen IF, Hillner BE, Hanna L, et al. Hospice admission and survival after ^{18}F-fluoride PET performed for evaluation of osseous metastatic disease in the national oncologic PET registry. J Nucl Med. 2018;59:427–33.
3. Oyen W, Sundram F, Haug AR, et al. Radium-223 dichloride (Ra-223) for the treatment of metastatic castration-resistant prostate cancer: optimizing clinical practice in nuclear medicine centers. J Oncopathol. 2015;3:1–25.
4. Sorto G, Gallichio R, Pellegrino T, et al. Impact of ^{18}F-fluoride PET/CT on implementing early treatment of painful bone metastases with Sm-153 EDTMP. Nucl Med Biol. 2013;40:518–23.
5. Even-Sapir E, Metser U, Mishani E, et al. The detection of bone metastases in patients with high-risk prostate cancer: ^{99m}Tc-MDP Planar bone scintigraphy; single- and multi-field-of-view SPECT; ^{18}F-fluoride PET; and [18]Ffluoride PET/CT. J Nucl Med. 2006;47:287–97.
6. Kairemo K, Milton DR, Etchebehere E, et al. Final outcome of [223]Ra-therapy and the role of ^{18}F-fluoride-PET in response evaluation in metastatic castration-resistant prostate cancer–a single institution experience. Curr Radiopharm. 2018;11:152–7.
7. Etchebehere EC, Araujo JC, Fox PS, Swanston NM, Macapinlac HA, Rohren EM. Prognostic factors in patients treated with 223Ra: the role of skeletal tumor turden on baseline [18]Ffluoride PET/CT in predicting overall survival. J Nucl Med. 2015;56:1177–84.
8. von Eyben FE, Kairemo K, Kiljunen T, Joensuu T. Planning of external beam radiotherapy for prostate cancer guided by PET/CT. Curr Radiopharm. 2015;8:19–31.
9. Hillner BE, Siegel BA, Hanna L, Duan F, Shields AF, Coleman RE. Impact of ^{18}F-fluoride PET in patients with known prostate cancer: initial results from the national oncologic PET registry. J Nucl Med. 2014;55:574–81.
10. Langsteger W, Balogova S, Huchet V, et al. Fluorocholine (^{18}F) and sodium fluoride (^{18}F) PET/CT in the detection of prostate cancer: prospective comparison of diagnostic performance determined by masked reading. Q J Nucl Med Mol Imaging. 2011;55:448–57.
11. Scher HI, Sawyers CL. Biology of progressive, castration resistant prostate cancer: directed therapies targeting the androgen receptor signaling axis. J Clin Oncol. 2005;23:8253–61.
12. Kairemo K, Joensuu T. Radium-223-dichloride in castration resistant metastatic prostate cancer-preliminary results of the response evaluation using F-18-fluoride PET/CT. Diagnostics (Basel). 2015;5:413–27.
13. Etchebehere E, Brito AE, Rezaee A, et al. Therapy assessment of bone metastatic disease in the era of [223]radium. Eur J Nucl Med Mol Imaging. 2017;44(Suppl 1):84–96.
14. Taube T, Elomaa I, Blomqvist C, Beneton MN, Kanis JA. Histomorphometric evidence for osteoclast-mediated bone resorption in metastatic breast cancer. Bone. 1994;15:161–6.

15. WAM B, van der Zant FM, Wondergem M, Knol RJJ. Accuracy of ^{18}F-NaF PET/CT in bone metastasis detection and its effect on patient management in patients with breast carcinoma. Nucl Med Commun. 2018;39(4):325–33.
16. Brito AE, Santos A, Sasse AD, et al. ^{18}F-Fluoride PET/CT tumor burden quantification predicts survival in breast cancer. Oncotarget. 2017;8(22):36001–11.
17. Azad G, Siddique MM, Taylor B, et al. Does measurement of ^{18}F-fluoride metabolic flux improve response assessment of breast cancer bone metastases compared with standardised uptake values in ^{18}F-fluoride PET/CT? J Nucl Med. 2019;60:322. https://doi.org/10.2967/jnumed.118.208710.
18. Peterson LM, O'Sullivan J, Wu QV, et al. Prospective study of serial ^{18}F-FDG PET and ^{18}F-fluoride (^{18}F-NaF) PET to predict time to skeletal related events, time-to-progression, and survival in patients with bone-dominant metastatic breast cancer. J Nucl Med. 2018;59:1823. https://doi.org/10.2967/jnumed.118.211102.
19. Rao L, Zong Z, Chen Z, et al. ^{18}F-labeled NaF PET/CT in detection of bone metastases in patients with preoperative lung cancer. Medicine (Baltimore). 2016;95:e3490.
20. Lee H, Lee WW, Park SY, Kim SE. F-18 sodium fluoride positron emission tomography/computed tomography for detection of thyroid cancer bone metastasis compared with bone scintigraphy. Korean J Radiol. 2016;17:281–8. https://doi.org/10.3348/kjr.2016.17.2.281.
21. Ota N, Kato K, Iwano S, et al. Comparison of ^{18}F-fluoride PET/CT, ^{18}F-FDG PET/CT and bone scintigraphy (planar and SPECT) in detection of bone metastases of differentiated thyroid cancer: a pilot study. Br J Radiol. 2014;87:20130444.
22. Schirrmeister H, Buck A, Guhlmann A, Reske SN. Anatomical distribution and sclerotic activity of bone metastases from thyroid cancer assessed with F-18 sodium fluoride positron emission tomography. Thyroid. 2001;11:677–83.
23. Gerety EL, Lawrence EM, Wason J, et al. Prospective study evaluating the relative sensitivity of ^{18}F-NaF PET/CT for detecting skeletal metastases from renal cell carcinoma in comparison to multidetector CT and 99mTc-MDP bone scintigraphy, using an adaptive trial design. Ann Oncol. 2015;26:2113–8.
24. Sharma P, Karunanithi S, Chakraborty PS, et al. ^{18}F-fluoride PET/CT for detection of bone metastasis in patients with renal cell carcinoma: a pilot study. Nucl Med Commun. 2014;35:1247–53.
25. Duarte PS, de Castroneves LA, Sado HN, et al. Bone and calcified soft tissue metastases of medullary thyroid carcinoma better characterized on ^{18}F-fluoride PET/CT than on ^{68}Ga-Dotatate PET/CT. Nucl Med Mol Imaging. 2018;52:318–23. https://doi.org/10.1007/s13139-018-0527-8.
26. Duarte PS, Marin JFG, Carvalho D, et al. Brain metastasis of medullary thyroid carcinoma without macroscopic calcification detected first on ^{68}Ga-Dotatate and then on ^{18}F-fluoride PET/CT. Clin Nucl Med. 2018;43:623–4.
27. do Vale RH, Marin JF, Duarte PS, Sapienza MT, Buchpiguel CA. Visualization of lymph nodal and hepatic metastases of medullary thyroid carcinoma on ^{18}F-fluoride PET/CT. Clin Nucl Med. 2015;40:895–6.
28. Basu S, Ranade R, Thapa P. ^{177}Lu-DOTATATE versus ^{177}Lu-EDTMP versus cocktail/sequential therapy in bone-confined painful metastatic disease in medullary carcinoma of the thyroid and neuroendocrine tumour: can semiquantitative comparison of ^{68}Ga-DOTATATE and ^{18}F-fluoride PET/CT aid in personalized treatment decision making in selecting the best therapeutic option? Nucl Med Commun. 2016;37:100–2.

¹⁸F-Fluoride Imaging: Monitoring Therapy

4

Elba Etchebehere and Kalevi Kairemo

Contents

4.1 Introduction

Novel oncologic therapeutic agents, whether chemotherapy, hormone therapy, immunotherapy, or radiotracers such as ^{223}Ra and ^{177}Lu-PSMA are expensive and diagnostic test able to predict and monitor response to treatment, avoid overtreatment and unnecessary costs, will improve patient management and guide individualized therapy.

E. Etchebehere (✉)
Division of Nuclear Medicine, University of Campinas (UNICAMP), Campinas, Brazil

K. Kairemo
Department of Nuclear Medicine and Molecular Radiotherapy, Docrates Cancer Center, Helsinki, Finland

© Springer Nature Switzerland AG 2020

27

K. Kairemo, H. A. Macapinlac (eds.), *Sodium Fluoride PET/CT in Clinical Use*, Clinicians' Guides to Radionuclide Hybrid Imaging, https://doi.org/10.1007/978-3-030-23577-2_4

Proper treatment of bone metastases requires adequate images. The morphology and extent of osteoblastic bone metastases, especially when widespread throughout the axial and appendicular skeleton, pose a challenge for conventional anatomic imaging (such as computed tomography and magnetic resonance imaging) to determine the tumor load and evaluate objectively response to therapy.

Conventional bone scintigraphy has been consistently proven to be an inaccurate and insensitive imaging tool to assess response to therapy in metastatic castration resistant prostate cancer (mCRPC). Only with unequivocal new lesions is there a benefit to monitoring therapy with conventional bone scan. Although conventional bone scintigraphy is capable of determining the extent of osteoblastic bone metastases, this imaging method is not a prognostic indicator because the exact extent of tumor load is underdiagnosed.

On the other hand, ^{18}F-Fluoride PET/CT has the ability to determine the full extent of bone tumor burden, is more accurate when compared to conventional bone scintigraphy, and has the advantage of permitting absolute quantification. Even though the evaluation of outcome prior to treatment and response after treatment is challenging and not fully well established with ^{18}F-Fluoride PET/CT, studies have consistently shown that objective quantification seems more promising to monitor therapy when compared to subjective image analysis [1].

Furthermore, a diagnostic radiotracer such as ^{18}F-Fluoride (a bone-seeking radiotracer for diagnosis) that has uptake properties similar to a therapeutic radiotracer such as [223]Ra (the bone-seeking radiotracer for therapy) has the potential to precisely assess the possibility and efficacy of a treatment (the *Theranostic* concept).

In this chapter, we will discuss ^{18}F-Fluoride PET/CT's capability to monitor therapy in three different time points: prior to initiation of therapy (baseline scans), during treatment (interim scans), and after therapy (follow-up scans).

4.2 Baseline ^{18}F-Fluoride PET/CT

[18]F-Fluoride PET/CT has superior sensitivity, specificity, and accuracy, when compared to other imaging modalities including PET/CT, bone scintigraphy with SPECT/CT, and whole-body MRI, to detect osteoblastic metastases in a variety of cancers [2–4]. This is noteworthy in cancers such as breast [5, 6], prostate [7], lung [8, 9], and renal cell carcinoma [10, 11]. Recently, ^{18}F-Fluoride PET/CT was shown to improve management of oral cavity cancers with suspicion on bone invasion. No modality was better than ^{18}F-Fluoride PET/CT (when compared to ^{18}F-FDG, CT or MRI) to determine the limits of mandibular tumor infiltration; in >85% of the patients studied, the difference of tumor extension by ^{18}F-Fluoride PET/CT compared to histology results were less than 10 mm [12].

[18]F-Fluoride PET/CT's higher spatial resolution lead to improved patient management because of the capability to determine, in a timely manner, the proper initial therapy in the early stages of cancers by detecting small osteoblastic metastases. If available, ^{18}F-Fluoride PET/CT should be the image of choice as it leads to improved patient management, as well as reduced waiting time to perform images when com-

pared to conventional bone scans [13]. Another potential advantage of 18F-Fluoride PET/CT is the concurrently acquired CT images, which enables the detection of soft tissue and/or visceral metastases, consequently increasing specificity.

In addition, baseline 18F-Fluoride PET/CT imaging has been shown to be a prognostic imaging biomarker, helpful in therapy monitoring. Many different parameters are being investigated, the vast majority in prostate cancer.

Below we will discuss 18F-Fluoride PET/CT's capability to monitor therapy in different cancer types.

4.2.1 Prostate Cancer

Osteoblastic bone metastases originating from prostate cancer may predominate or be the only site of disease. The assessment of prognosis prior to and during treatment of prostate cancer is crucial to increase the odds of individualized patient management and of better outcome.

Retrospective and prospective studies have shown that the whole-body skeletal tumor burden on baseline 18F-Fluoride PET/CT is a powerful imaging biomarker, capable of independently evaluating prognosis in prostate cancer patients [14, 15]. The calculation of skeletal tumor burden on baseline 18F-Fluoride PET/CT has been conducted by establishing basically two different SUVmax thresholds: SUVmax = 10 [16] and SUVmax = 15 [17]. Regardless of the quantification method and the threshold levels described above, all are reproducible and have a remarkable prognostic power [18]. *Please refer to Chap. 5 for the step-by-step method on the quantification of bone tumor burden on 18F-fluoride in PET/CT.*

Baseline 18F-Fluoride PET/CT estimation of tumor burden may be able to define which prostate cancer patients will benefit from 223Ra therapy. 223Ra is a bone-seeking therapeutic radionuclide that increases overall survival in metastatic castrate-resistant prostate cancer (mCRPC) patients [19]. The 18F-fluoride uptake in osteoblastic bone metastases from prostate cancer measured in baseline 18F-Fluoride PET/CT images has been shown to strongly, significantly, and directly correlate with the corresponding uptake and absorbed dose of 223Ra, and these metrics can help evaluate subsequent lesion response to treatment [20, 21]. Additionally, 18F-Fluoride PET/CT is useful in patients with end-stage disease to monitor the odds of developing bone marrow failure after 223Ra due to extensive bone marrow tumor infiltration [22].

4.2.2 Breast Cancer

The skeleton is the major site of distant metastases in breast cancer patients although, unlike prostate cancer, osteolytic and osteoblastic lesions are present. Even though osteolytic lesions may be present in breast cancer patients, 18F-Fluoride uptake occurs in these osteolytic lesions because of the surrounding osteoblastic response.

Monitoring therapy in breast cancer can also be achieved by calculating the skeletal tumor burden on ^{18}F-Fluoride PET/CT [23]. Most importantly, the determination of the skeletal tumor burden in ^{18}F-Fluoride PET/CT images has been shown to be an independent imaging biomarker of prognosis in these patients. This information will lead to proper patient management as there are no laboratory or other imaging biomarkers that, in disease that has affected the skeleton, can independently assess the outcome to determine the adequate treatment strategy [24].

4.3 Interim ^{18}F-Fluoride PET/CT

The ideal moment to perform ^{18}F-Fluoride PET/CT scan to assess response to treatment is quite unclear. Bone restoration as a consequence of appropriate treatment causes an osteoblastic reaction in order to restore normal bone, increasing ^{18}F-Fluoride uptake, which is known as a flare response [25]. Flare responses may occur as early as the first cycle of therapy, whether with [223]Ra for prostate cancer [26] or chemotherapy, monoclonal antibody therapy [27], or hormonal therapy for breast cancer [28]. The flare phenomenon generally peaks and diminishes approximately 2 months after initiation of therapy. This may explain why ^{18}F-fluoride PET/CT scans performed 3 months after the beginning of therapy is a more reliable measure of tumor response than scans acquired after 2 months [29].

Unfortunately, progression of osteoblastic bone metastases will also cause an increase in osteoblastic reaction and inflammation secondary to tumor-associated growth factors. Therefore the occurrence of the flare phenomenon reduces the specificity of interim scans to determine response to therapy. Even though the CT portion of the ^{18}F-Fluoride PET/CT scans normally reveals reparative changes noted by the increased extent of the sclerotic lesions, there is no guarantee that this phenomenon is due to reparative changes and not due to progressive disease.

4.3.1 Prostate Cancer

Interim ^{18}F-Fluoride PET/CT scans have been performed in prostate cancer patients in the advanced stages as well as in the early stages of cancer. Kairemo et al. initially published *a small series of 10 mCRPC patients submitted to* interim ^{18}F-Fluoride PET/CT scans and demonstrated that the determination of outcome after [223]Ra was not possible since increased uptake was noted in responders and in non-responders [30]. *They further confirmed these preliminary results* in a larger population ($n = 161$) submitted to 772 [223]Ra cycles [31].

Likewise, Etchebehere et al. [32] evaluated 68 ^{18}F-Fluoride PET/CT scans of mCRPC submitted to [223]Ra therapy to determine if the interim scan could predict overall survival, progression-free survival, or time to a skeletal-related event. None of those outcome measures could be determined by interim ¹⁸F-Fluoride PET/CT scans. Additionally, in their study, a finding not described before in the literature was the decrease in ¹⁸F-Fluoride uptake on the interim scan compared to the baseline scan in a small group of patients that developed bone marrow failure due to extensive bone marrow infiltration by tumor. On the contrary, in other patients, the increased ¹⁸F-Fluoride uptake was due to a flare phenomenon, posing a difficulty in determining which patients were progressing and which were responding. In their study, bone ALP levels had higher specificity than the interim ¹⁸F-Fluoride PET/CT scan.

However, while an interim ¹⁸F-Fluoride PET/CT scan may not be useful to determine outcome after ²²³Ra therapy, its use on various chemotherapeutic, tyrosine kinase, and hormonal agents may be impactful. For example, changes in interim ¹⁸F-Fluoride PET/CT scans to determine response to dasatinib therapy in 12 mCRPC have been shown to correlate well with bone alkaline phosphatase levels but have a borderline correlation with progression-free survival [33]. Contrary to expected findings, the mCRPC patients with the largest decrease in ¹⁸F-Fluoride uptake within the osteoblastic metastases in response to dasatinib had the worst outcomes while those patients with a lower decline or even an increase in osteoblastic activity had the longest duration of therapy until progression. This may be caused by the properties of dasatinib, promoting osteoblast differentiation and activation, thus increasing bone mineralization, comparable to a flare phenomenon seen on ¹⁸F-fluoride PET/CT scans.

In mCRPC patients undergoing chemotherapy or hormonal therapy, a recent study evaluated the ability of baseline and interim (after three cycles of therapy) ¹⁸F-Fluoride PET/CT scans to determine outcome of androgen receptor pathway inhibitors (*n* = 40) and chemotherapy (*n* = 16) in 56 mCRPC patients with osteoblastic metastases. The interim ¹⁸F-Fluoride PET/CT scan was the strongest univariable predictor of progression-free survival [34].

These different studies have demonstrated that the variation of ¹⁸F-Fluoride uptake may be associated with the mechanism of therapeutic reaction within the bone. For example, bone-activating agents (such as ²²³Ra and dasatinib) may promote a flare response, and thus the increased ¹⁸F-Fluoride uptake may be related to better outcome. Quite the reverse, when using therapeutic agents that do not promote bone-activation (such as chemotherapy and hormonal therapy agents), the increase in ¹⁸F-Fluoride uptake may be related to worst outcome.

Therefore, it is not possible to extrapolate the ¹⁸F-Fluoride uptake results obtained from the evaluation of one drug to all forms of systemic therapy, including secondary hormone therapy, chemotherapy, radiation therapy, monoclonal antibodies, and osteoclast activating inhibitors. The mechanism of action of individual drugs may vary and the differences in biological behavior of tumor types and effects on the skeleton may also differ.

An evaluation at 12 weeks after initiation of systemic therapy for bone metastases remains at an early enough time point to be clinically relevant in informing clinical management decisions and for measuring early response in clinical trials (Figs. 4.1 and 4.2).

a   b

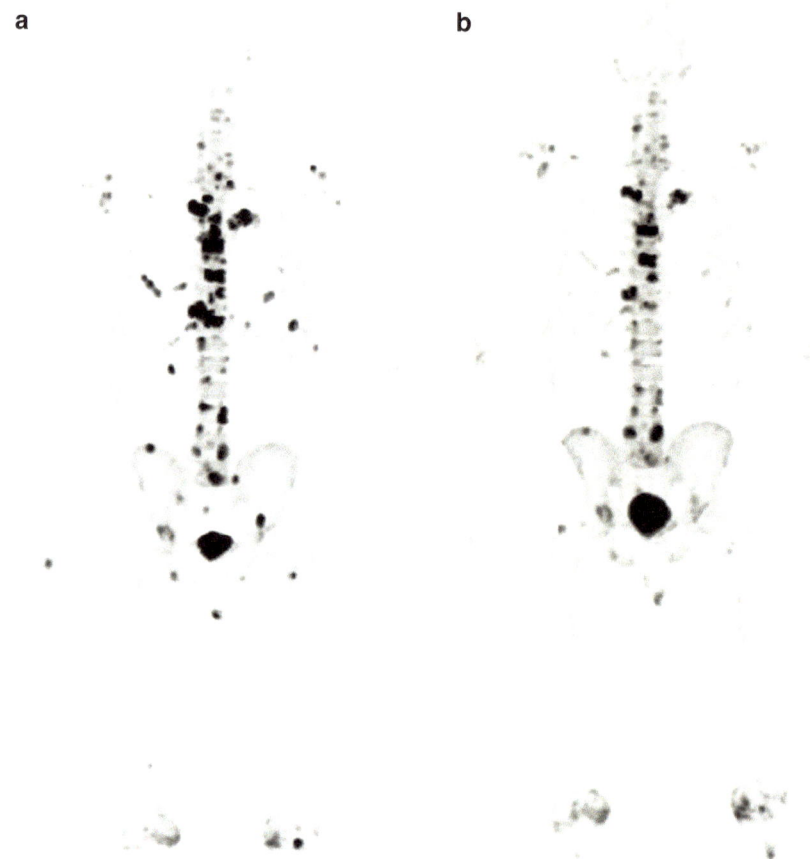

Fig. 4.1 ^{18}F-Fluoride PET/CT baseline (a) and interim (b) scans of a mCRPC patient submitted to [223]Ra. The (a) baseline ^{18}F-Fluoride PET/CT scan shows widespread osteoblastic metastases. The (b) interim ^{18}F-Fluoride PET/CT scan performed after the third [223]Ra cycle demonstrates reduction of osteoblastic metastases especially in the rib cages, pelvis, and right femur, consistent with partial response to [223]Ra

4.3.2 Breast Cancer

There are a limited number of studies evaluating the role of interim ^{18}F-Fluoride PET/CT to determine response to therapy in metastatic breast cancer patients.

In one study, the ^{18}F-fluoride metabolic flux (Ki) measurement calculated after 8 weeks of endocrine treatment for bone-predominant metastatic breast cancer seems more reliable in differentiating progressive disease from nonprogressive disease when compared to semi-quantitative SUV measures. The Ki was better than quantitative SUV measurements since the SUV metrics in general underestimates

a   b

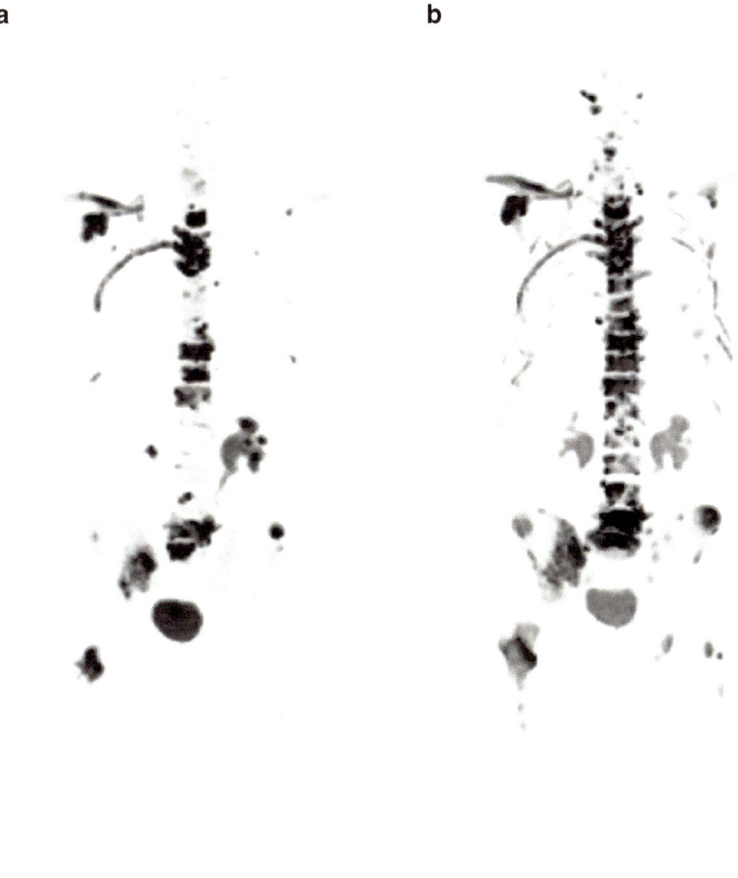

Fig. 4.2 ¹⁸F-Fluoride PET/CT baseline (**a**) and interim (**b**) scans of a mCRPC patient submitted to ²²³Ra. The (**a**) baseline ¹⁸F-Fluoride PET/CT scan shows widespread osteoblastic metastases. The (**b**) interim ¹⁸F-Fluoride PET/CT scan performed after the third ²²³Ra cycle demonstrates increase in the number of osteoblastic metastases, consistent with progression while on ²²³Ra

the ¹⁸F-Fluoride clearance from metastatic bone. These initial results, observed in 12 patients, need further prospective validation in larger patient groups under different therapy regimes [35].

Dynamic ¹⁸F-Fluoride PET/CT studies demonstrate a decrease of kinetic parameters as response to treatment, reflecting changes at a molecular level before any morphological modifications arise.

4.4   Follow-Up ^{18}F-Fluoride PET/CT

4.4.1   Prostate Cancer

Unlike the use of interim ^{18}F-Fluoride PET/CT to monitor therapy in which uptake may vary and depend on the type of therapy being applied, the use of ^{18}F-Fluoride PET/CT at the end of therapy has demonstrated better results.

Kairemo et al. performed ^{18}F-Fluoride PET/CT images at baseline and 6 weeks after the last ^{223}Ra cycle in 10 mCRPC patients. A quantitative reduction of ^{18}F-Fluoride uptake ranging from 7% to 68% was noted in all patients that responded to ^{223}Ra treatment [30]. *The quantitative assessment of* ^{18}F-Fluoride PET/CT was based on modified PET-response criteria, i.e., the sum of the SUVs from two regions [30]. The total skeletal burden such as TLF_{10} [14, Chap. 5] is more precise in the follow-up setting. The study which analyzed ^{18}F-Fluoride PET/CT scans to determine outcome of androgen receptor pathway inhibitors ($n = 40$) and chemotherapy ($n = 16$) in mCRPC patients with osseous metastases used actually TLF_{15} as a disease indicator and it turned out to be the strongest parameter to predict progression-free survival [34].

A recent study compared the accuracy of a first generation ^{18}F-labelled prostate-specific membrane antigen (PSMA)-targeted agent (^{18}F-DCFBC PET/CT) and of ^{18}F-Fluoride PET/CT to evaluate treatment response of 28 mCRPC patients submitted to androgen deprivation therapy. In patients on androgen deprivation therapy with early or metastatic castrate sensitive disease (PSA levels below 2 ng/ml), follow-up images after androgen deprivation therapy demonstrated significantly more lesions (residual disease) on ^{18}F-Fluoride PET/CT compared to ^{18}F-DCFBC. However, in patients with advanced mCRPC, the residual number of bone lesions was similar or higher on ^{18}F-DCFBC compared to ^{18}F-Fluoride PET/CT. Therefore the utility of each radiotracer will depend on patient disease course and treatment status [36].

4.4.2   Breast Cancer

A study conducted on 28 patients with breast cancer and metastases to the bone were evaluated with ^{18}F-Fluoride PET/CT performed at a baseline and approximately 4 months after initiation of therapy. The increase in the ^{18}F-Fluoride uptake between scans was associated with longer overall survival, although they were not predictive of time-to skeletal-related events or to time-to-progression [23].

4.4.3   Multiple Myeloma

In multiple myeloma patients, ^{18}F-Fluoride PET/CT scans do not seem to add significantly to response to therapy. A study evaluating the benefit of ^{18}F-Fluoride PET/CT for treatment response assessment of multiple myeloma in 34 patients undergoing high-dose chemotherapy followed by autologous stem cell transplantation showed that, even though 65% of the patients responded to treatment, 85% of the follow-up ^{18}F-Fluoride PET/CT images were unaltered compared to of baseline images [37].

4.5 Conclusion

^{18}F-Fluoride PET/CT seems promising in the assessment of therapy as a prognostic imaging biomarker. Quantitative approach by defining skeletal tumor burden provides more accurate assessment of prognosis and response to therapy. Optimal disease evaluation by ^{18}F-Fluoride PET/CT imaging can be performed at baseline, at interim, or at the end of therapy, depending on the therapeutic regimen.

In order to properly evaluate response to treatment, it seems reasonable to prefer quantification analyses to subjective qualitative reading to reduce reader-dependent subjectivity, inter- and intra-observer variability, to detect subtle tumor regression or progression, and to obtain objective measures of bone metastases response.

References

1. Lin C, Bradshaw T, Perk T, Harmon S, Eickhoff J, Jallow N, et al. Repeatability of quantitative ^{18}F-NaF PET: a multicenter study. J Nucl Med. 2016;57:1872–9.
2. Bortot DC, Amorim BJ, Oki GC, Gapski SB, Santos AO, Lima MC, et al. ^{18}F-fluoride PET/CT is highly effective for excluding bone metastases even in patients with equivocal bone scintigraphy. Eur J Nucl Med Mol Imaging. 2012;39:1730–6.
3. Shen C, Qiu Z, Han T, Luo Q. Performance of ^{18}F-fluoride PET or PET/CT for the detection of bone metastases. A meta-analysis. Clin Nucl Med. 2015;40:103–10.
4. Minamimoto R, Loening A, Jamali M, Barkhodari A, Mosci C, Jackson T, et al. Prospective comparison of 99mTc-MDP scintigraphy, combined ^{18}F-NaF and ^{18}F-FDG PET/CT, and whole-body MRI in patients with breast and prostate cancer. J Nucl Med. 2015;56:1862–8.
5. Abikhzer G, Srour S, Fried G, Drumea K, Kozlener E, Frenkel A, et al. Prospective comparison of whole-body bone SPECT and sodium ^{18}F-fluoride PET in the detection of bone metastases from breast cancer. Nucl Med Commun. 2016;37:1160–8.
6. Broos W, van der Zant FM, Wondergem M, Knol RJJ. Accuracy of ^{18}F-NaF PET/CT in bone metastasis detection and its effect on patient management in patients with breast carcinoma. Nucl Med Commun. 2018;39:325–33.
7. Even-Sapir E, Metser U, Mishani E, Lievshitz G, Lerman H, Leibovitch I. The detection of bone metastases in patients with high-risk prostate cancer: 99mTc-MDP planar bone scintigraphy, single- and multi-field-of-view SPECT, ^{18}F-fluoride PET, and ^{18}F-fluoride PET/CT. J Nucl Med. 2006;47:287–97.
8. Kruger S, Buck AK, Mottaghy FM, Hasenkamp E, Pauls S, Schumann C, et al. Detection of bone metastases in patients with lung cancer: 99mTc-MDP planar bone scintigraphy, ^{18}F-fluoride PET or ^{18}F-FDG PET/CT. Eur J Nucl Med Mol Imaging. 2009;36:1807–12.
9. Rao L, Zong Z, Chen Z, Wang X, Shi X, Yi C, et al. ^{18}F-labeled NaF PET/CT in detection of bone metastases in patients with preoperative lung cancer. Medicine. 2016;95:e3490.
10. Sharma P, Karunanithi S, Chakraborty PS, Kumar R, Seth A, Julka PK, Bal C, Kumar R. ^{18}F-fluoride PET/CT for detection of bone metastasis in patients with renal cell carcinoma: a pilot study. Nucl Med Commun. 2014;35:1247–53.

11. Gerety EL, Lawrence EM, Wason J, Yan H, Hilborne S, Buscombe J, et al. Prospective study evaluating the relative sensitivity of ^{18}F-NaF PET/CT for detecting skeletal metastases from renal cell carcinoma in comparison to multidetector CT and 99mTc-MDP bone scintigraphy, using an adaptive trial design. Ann Oncol. 2015;26:2113–8.

12. Lopez R, Gantet P, Salabert AS, Julian A, Hitzel A, Herbault-Barres B, Fontan C, Alshehri S, Payoux P. Prospective comparison of ^{18}F-NaF PET/CT versus ^{18}F-FDG PET/CT imaging in mandibular extension of head and neck squamous cell carcinoma with dedicated analysis software and validation with surgical specimen. A preliminary study. J Craniomaxillofac Surg. 2017;45:1486–92.

13. Hillner BE, Siegel BA, Hanna L, Duan F, Quinn B, Shields AF. ^{18}F-fluoride PET used for treatment monitoring of systemic cancer therapy: results from the national oncologic PET registry. J Nucl Med. 2015;56:222–8.

14. Etchebehere EC, Araujo JC, Fox PS, Swanston NM, Macapinlac HA, Rohren EM. Prognostic factors in patients treated with 223Ra: the role of skeletal tumor burden on baseline ^{18}F-fluoride PET/CT in predicting overall survival. J Nucl Med. 2015;56:1177–84.

15. Apolo AB, Lindenberg L, Shih JH, Mena E, Kim JW, Park JC, et al. Prospective study evaluating Na[18]F PET/CT in predicting clinical outcomes and survival in advanced prostate cancer. J Nucl Med. 2016;57:886–92.

16. Rohren EM, Etchebehere EC, Araujo JC, Hobbs BP, Swanston NM, Everding M, et al. Determination of skeletal tumor burden on ^{18}F-fluoride PET/CT. J Nucl Med. 2015;56: 1507–12.

17. Lindgren B, Sadik M, Kaboteh R, Hasani N, Enqvist O, Svärm L, Kahl F, Simonsen J, Poulsen M, Ohlsson M, Høilund-Carlsen P, Edenbrandt L, Trägårdh E. 3D skeletal uptake of ^{18}F sodium fluoride in PET/CT images is associated with overall survival in patients with prostate cancer. EJNMMI Res. 2017;7:15.

18. Lin C, Bradshaw T, Perk T, Harmon S, Eickhoff J, Jallow N, Choyke PL, Dahut WL, Larson S, Humm JL, Perlman S, Apolo AB, Morris MJ, Liu G, Jeraj R. Repeatability of quantitative ^{18}F-NaF PET: a multicenter study. J Nucl Med. 2016;57:1872–9.

19. Parker C, Nilsson S, Heinrich D, Helle SI, O'Sullivan JM, Fossa SD, et al. Alpha emitter radium-223 and survival in metastatic prostate cancer. N Engl J Med. 2013;369:213–23.

20. Letellier A, Johnson AC, Kit NH, Savigny J, Batalla A, Parienti J, Aide N. Uptake of radium-223 dichloride and early [^{18}F] NaF PET response are driven by baseline [^{18}F]NaF parameters: a pilot study in castration-resistant prostate cancer patients. Mol Imaging Biol. 2018;20:482–91.

21. Murray I, Chittenden SJ, Denis-Bacelar AM, Hindorf C, Parker C, Chua S, Flux GD. The potential of 223Ra and ^{18}F-fluoride imaging to predict bone lesion response to treatment with 223Ra-dichloride in castration-resistant prostate cancer. Eur J Nucl Med Mol Imaging. 2017;44:1832–44.

22. Etchebehere EC, Araujo JC, Milton DR, Erwin WD, Wendt RE 3rd, Swanston NM, et al. Skeletal tumor burden on baseline ^{18}F-fluoride PET/CT predicts bone marrow failure after 223Ra therapy. Clin Nucl Med. 2016;41:268–73.

23. Peterson LM, O'Sullivan J, Wu QV, Novakova-Jiresova A, Jenkins I, Lee JH, Shields A, Montgomery S, Linden HM, Gralow JR, Gadi VK, Muzi M, Kinahan PE, Mankoff DA, Specht JM. Prospective study of serial ^{18}F-FDG PET and ^{18}F-fluoride (^{18}F-NaF) PET to predict time to skeletal related events, time-to-progression, and survival in patients with bone-dominant metastatic breast cancer. J Nucl Med. 2018;59:1823. https://doi.org/10.2967/jnumed.118.211102.

24. Brito A, Santos A, Sasse AD, Cabello C, Oliveira P, Mosci C, Souza T, Amorim B, Lima M, Ramos CD, Etchebehere E. ^{18}F-Fluoride PET/CT tumor burden quantification predicts survival in breast cancer. Oncotarget. 2017;8:36001–11.

25. Rossleigh MA, Lovegrove FT, Reynolds PM, Byrne MJ. Serial bone scans in the assessment of response to therapy in advanced breast carcinoma. Clin Nucl Med. 1982;7:397–402.

26. Castello A, Macapinlac HA, Lopci E, Santos EB. Prostate-specific antigen flare induced by 223RaCl2 in patients with metastatic castration-resistant prostate cancer. Eur J Nucl Med Mol Imaging. 2018;45:2256. https://doi.org/10.1007/s00259-018-4051-y. [Epub ahead of print].

27. Balasubramanian Harisankar CN, Preethi R, John J. Metabolic flare phenomenon on 18 fluoride-fluorodeoxy glucose positron emission tomography-computed tomography scans in a patient with bilateral breast cancer treated with second-line chemotherapy and bevacizumab. Indian J Nucl Med. 2015;30:145–7.
28. Wade AA, Scott JA, Kuter I, Fischman AJ. Flare response in ^{18}F-fluoride ion PET bone scanning. AJR Am J Roentgenol. 2006;186:1783–6.
29. Cook G Jr, Parker C, Chua S, Johnson B, Aksnes AK, Lewington VJ. ^{18}F-fluoride PET: changes in uptake as a method to assess response in bone metastases from castrate-resistant prostate cancer patients treated with 223Ra-chloride (Alpharadin). EJNMMI Res. 2011;1:4.
30. Kairemo K, Joensuu T. Radium-223-dichloride in castration resistant metastatic prostate cancer-preliminary results of the response evaluation using F-18-fluoride PET/CT. Diagnostics. 2015;5:413–27.
31. Kairemo K, Milton DR, Etchebehere E, Rohren EM, Macapinlac HA. Final outcome of 223Ra-therapy and the role of ^{18}F-fluoride-PET in response evaluation in metastatic castration resistant prostate cancer—a single institution experience. Curr Radiopharm. 2018;11:147–52.
32. Etchebehere E, Brito AE, Kairemo K, Araujo J, Rohren E, Macapinlac H. Interim ^{18}F-fluoride PET/CT is not able to predict outcome after radium-223 therapy. Radiol Bras. 2019;52:33.
33. Yu EY, Duan F, Muzi M, Deng X, Chin BB, Alumkal JJ, et al. Castration-resistant prostate cancer bone metastasis response measured by ^{18}F-fluoride PET after treatment with dasatinib and correlation with progression-free survival: results from American College of Radiology Imaging Network 6687. J Nucl Med. 2015;56:354–60.
34. Harmon SA, Perk T, Lin C, Eickhoff J, Choyke PL, Dahut WL, Apolo AB, Humm JL, Larson SM, Morris MJ, Liu G, Jeraj R. Quantitative assessment of early [^{18}F] sodium fluoride positron emission tomography/computed tomography response to treatment in men with metastatic prostate cancer to bone. J Clin Oncol. 2017;35:2829–37.
35. Azad GK, Siddique M, Taylor B, Green A, O'Doherty J, Gariani J, Blake GM, Mansi J, Goh V, Cook G. Is Response Assessment of Breast Cancer Bone Metastases Better with Measurement of ^{18}F-Fluoride Metabolic Flux Than with Measurement of ^{18}F-Fluoride PET/CT SUV? J Nucl Med. 2019;60:322–7.
36. Harmon SA, Bergvall E, Mena E, Shih JH, Adler S, McKinney Y, Mehralivand S, Citrin DE, Couvillon A, Madan R, Gulley J, Mease RC, Jacobs PM, Pomper MG, Turkbey B, Choyke PL, Lindenberg ML. A prospective comparison of ^{18}F-sodium fluoride PET/CT and PSMA-targeted ^{18}F-DCFBC PET/CT in metastatic prostate cancer. J Nucl Med. 2018;59:1665. https://doi.org/10.2967/jnumed.117.207373. [Epub ahead of print].
37. Sachpekidis C, Hillengass J, Goldschmidt H, Wagner B, Haberkorn U, Kopka K, Dimitrakopoulou-Strauss A. Treatment response evaluation with ^{18}F-FDG PET/CT and ^{18}F-NaF PET/CT in multiple myeloma patients undergoing high-dose chemotherapy and autologous stem cell transplantation. Eur J Nucl Med Mol Imaging. 2017;44:50–62.

Determination of Skeletal Tumor Burden on ^{18}F-Fluoride PET/CT

5

Ana Emília Brito and Elba Etchebehere

Contents

5.1 Introduction

Since first proposed in 1999 by Larson et al. [1], the use of volumetric quantification techniques on PET/CT exams has become increasingly popular to evaluate tumor burden, especially with ^{18}F-FDG. The volumetric quantification of tumor burden has been shown to correlate with prognosis and is also an objective means to evaluate response to treatment in a variety of cancers [2].

Skeletal tumor burden is obtained by volumetric quantification of ^{18}F-fluoride PET/CT studies. In summary, to obtain the skeletal tumor burden, initially, one must measure the mean total volume of all ^{18}F-fluoride bone-avid lesions, in milliliters

A. E. Brito
Real Nuclear, Real Hospital Português de Beneficência em Pernambuco, Recife, Brazil

E. Etchebehere (✉)
Division of Nuclear Medicine, University of Campinas (UNICAMP), Campinas, Brazil

© Springer Nature Switzerland AG 2020
K. Kairemo, H. A. Macapinlac (eds.), *Sodium Fluoride PET/CT in Clinical Use*,
Clinicians' Guides to Radionuclide Hybrid Imaging,
https://doi.org/10.1007/978-3-030-23577-2_5

(ml), also known as Fluoride Tumor Volume (FTV). Secondly, by adding the FTV metrics with the amount of ^{18}F-fluoride bone-avid lesions, measured in grams (g), the Total Lesion with ^{18}F-Fluoride uptake (TLF) is obtained.

In this chapter, we will discuss the clinical relevance of Skeletal Tumor Burden quantification and teach the reader how to perform volumetric quantification in ^{18}F-fluoride PET/CT studies both manually and semi-automatically.

5.2 Clinical Relevance and Rational to Determine the Skeletal Tumor Burden

The Volumetric Quantification of Skeletal Tumor Burden on ^{18}F-fluoride PET/CT has been performed mainly in prostate cancer since osteoblastic bone metastases are a strong determinant of survival in these patients. Furthermore, the recent use of radium-223 dichloride ([223]Ra) to treat osteoblastic bone metastases opens the possibility to evaluate the extent of ^{18}F-fluoride-avid bone metastases prior to therapy.

Studies have shown that the skeletal tumor burden on ^{18}F-fluoride PET/CT (quantified as TLF_{10}, i.e., using the SUVmax threshold of 10 for quantification) could predict survival [3] and predict the odds of developing bone marrow failure after [223]Ra [4]. Furthermore, Volumetric Quantification of Skeletal Tumor Burden has major advantages when compared to bone quantification in conventional bone scintigraphy. Even though in the latter quantification can be obtained, it has not been shown to be observer-independent or repeatable, correlating to biochemical variations in prostate cancer. On the other hand, on ^{18}F-fluoride PET/CT, even when using an SUV cut-off value of 15 to exclude more effectively degenerative bone changes [5], the results are reproducible.

In breast cancer patients, three studies have determined the skeletal tumor burden on ^{18}F-Fluoride PET/CT using a threshold of SUVmax = 10 [6–8]. The first two studies showed that ^{18}F-fluoride PET/CT skeletal tumor burden an independent prognostic imaging biomarker of overall survival and progression-free survival in 49 patients [6]. Additionally, the latter study demonstrated outstanding intra-observer and inter-observer reproducibility and that the percentage of the skeletal tumor burden variation in response to therapy (in 10 breast cancer patients) had a direct correlation with the percentage variation of the tumor markers.

Although there is a variety of quantification software available, so far only one study [7] has validated the semiautomatic ^{18}F-fluoride PET/CT quantification of the skeletal tumor burden; in 51 breast cancer patients there was a strong correlation with manual calculation and also with overall survival [7].

Next, we will demonstrate the step-by-step quantification process both manually and semi-automatically.

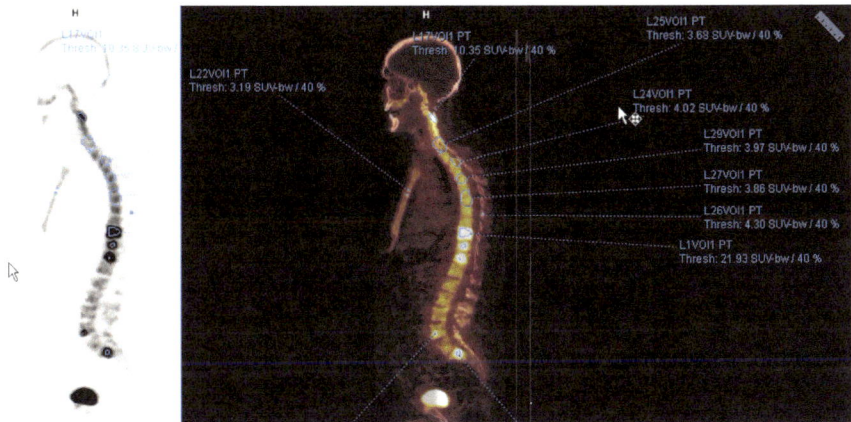

Fig. 5.1 An example of a patient with multiple ^{18}F-Fluoride-avid bone metastases. Volumes of interest were manually placed in all osteoblastic metastases in order to calculate the skeletal tumor burden. In patients such as this one, with a high bone tumor load, manual quantification process is difficult and time-consuming. Furthermore, it is an observer-dependent process, leading to a low reproducibility

5.3 ^{18}F-Fluoride PET/CT Manual Quantification

Manual quantification of the skeletal tumor burden on ^{18}F-Fluoride PET/CT studies is laborious. Manual recording of SUVmax and volume values of all ^{18}F-Fluoride bone metastases is necessary to calculate skeletal tumor burden. This is not possible in the daily routine due to the extent of bone metastases in some patients. The newer versions of PET/CT oncology software supply the FTV and TLF metrics once all VOIs are manually drawn.

In order to begin, initially upload the DICOM images to the quantification platform. The platform is necessary to calculate the standardized uptake values.

Second, identify all ^{18}F-Fluoride-avid metastatic bone lesions. Due to the excellent target-to-background ratio (osteoblastic metastases *versus* the normal skeleton), these lesions are easily noted [9, 10]. In this case, it is important to verify that only neoplastic areas are selected. Afterward, a 3D ellipsoid volume of interest (VOI) should be manually drawn surrounding all ^{18}F-Fluoride-avid bone metastases. It is important to define the isocontour threshold of these VOIs since the use of a smaller threshold increases the VOI´s volume and a larger threshold reduces the VOI´s volume. A threshold value used in practice and recommended by guidelines is 41% of the SUVmax [11]. The maximum SUV (SUVmax) and the volume (in milliliters) of each VOI should be annotated. The sum of all VOIs surrounding ^{18}F-Fluoride-avid bone metastases provides the FTV, which corresponds to the tumor volume (in milliliters). The TLF is the FTV value multiplied by the average of all SUVmax [12] (Fig. 5.1).

$$TLF = FTV \times average \ of \ all \ SUVmax$$

5.4 ^{18}F-Fluoride PET/CT Semi-Automatic Quantification

Semi-automatic quantification should be performed either on a PET/CT workstation with the quantification tool available or by exporting the DICOM images into a specific software program. The semi-automatic quantification will provide the same parameters described in the manual quantification (FTV and TFL), with the difference that it is not necessary to draw the VOIs manually nor perform all the calculations.

Initially, it is necessary to establish a cut-off SUVmax value to surround fluoride-avid metastases and exclude the normal bone. The SUVmax cut-off values most used are 10 and 15. Investigators quantified the spine, pelvic bones, and right femur of 142 ^{18}F-fluoride PET/CT scans and concluded that an SUVmax cut-off of 10 is sufficient to exclude the normal bone uptake from all required segmentations in 98% of the patients [12]. Two studies performed semi-automatic quantification of ^{18}F-fluoride PET/CT scans in 10 and 35 prostate cancer patients and established the SUVmax threshold of 15. Both studies concluded that TLF$_{15}$ correlated with PSA and ALP levels and found that this cut-off value was better to exclude more effectively degenerative bone changes and did not exclude any malignant lesion [5, 13].

Secondly, the quantification software should automatically generate a VOI surrounding the whole-body image. Afterward, select the SUVmax threshold (for example, SUVmax = 10) to allow the software to surround all regions with a SUVmax above the established threshold. At this point, it is important to review all the generated VOIs to exclude physiological uptakes (such as urinary tract and bladder), degenerative processes, and benign bone lesions, which could have high uptake.

A study evaluating the variation of SUV in patients with prostate cancer showed that the degenerative lesions present lower SUV values than metastatic lesions (11.1 ± 3.8 for degenerative lesions and 16.3 ± 13 for metastatic lesions); however, they present a wide variation and overlap of values [9]. Thus, review of all images is important regardless of the SUVmax value chosen.

Because of the necessity of manual exclusion, the quantification is not yet fully automatic. However, there are some studies showing experimental models of fully automatic volumetric quantification that exclude the need for segmentation and manual intervention [14]. Although they present good results in phantoms, clinical validation is still necessary.

After excluding all areas not related to fluoride-avid bone metastases, the software program will provide the FTV$_{10}$ and TLF$_{10}$ or FTV$_{15}$ and TLF $_{15}$ values, depending on the threshold established.

This process is fast and thus quantification can be incorporated into the routine clinical practice (Fig. 5.2).

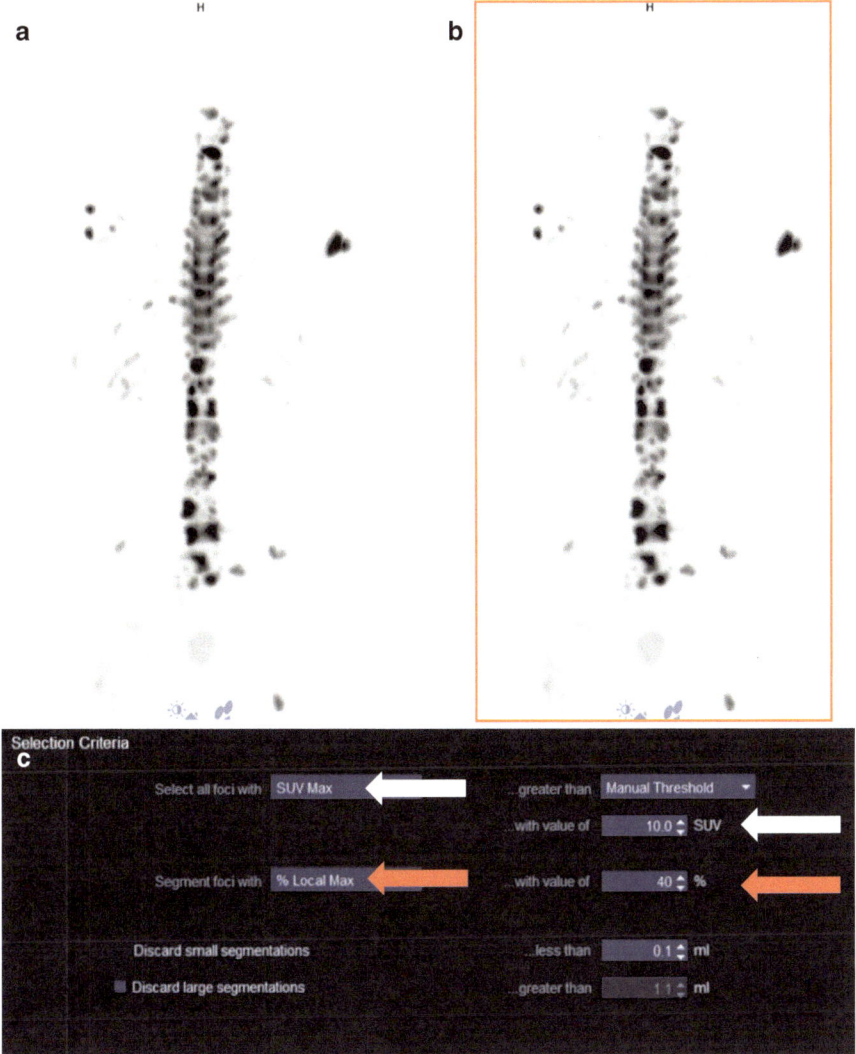

Fig. 5.2 (**a**) An example of calculation of the skeletal tumor burden on ^{18}F-Fluoride PET/CT scan in a patient with multiple widespread ^{18}F-Fluoride-avid bone metastases. Initially, careful diagnosis of all metastases and normal fluoride-avid uptake should be identified. (**b**) In order to perform quantification, initially a volume of interest (VOI) is semi-automatically drawn surrounding the MIP image (*red rectangle*). (**c**) Afterwards, select the quantification criteria that will be applied to the region within the VOI, such as the SUVmax threshold (*white arrows*) and the %threshold for each VOI (*red arrows*). In this particular case an SUVmax threshold of 10 and a 41% VOI threshold were established in order to separate all metastases from normal bone. (**d**) Then, the software will automatically generate multiple VOIs surrounding all the metastases, and the uptake in the normal bone structures is excluded from the multiple VOIs that are generated. At this point, careful evaluation and exclusion of any and all fluoride-avid regions not related to metastases should be performed. (**e**) The multiple VOIs provide the quantification parameters for each lesion. (**f**) The software will then generate the quantification parameters of whole-body tumor burden (FTV$_{10}$ and TLF$_{10}$). Even in patients such as this one, with a high bone tumor load, the semi-automatic quantification process is easy, fast, observer-independent, and highly reproducible (*white arrow*)

d   **e**

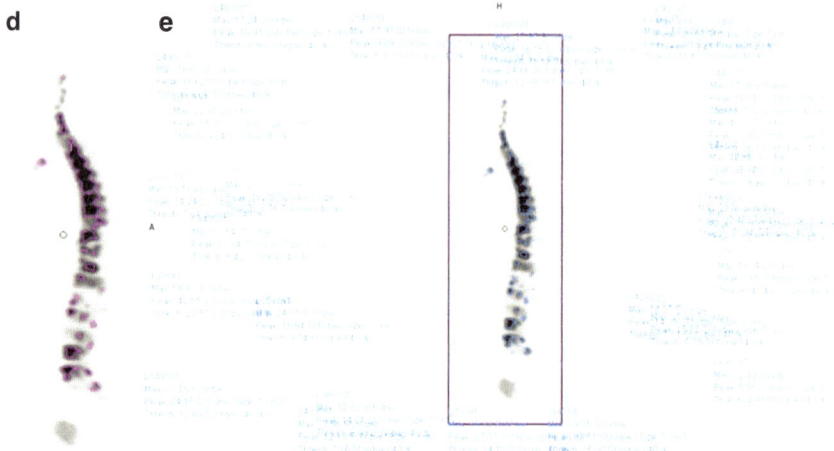

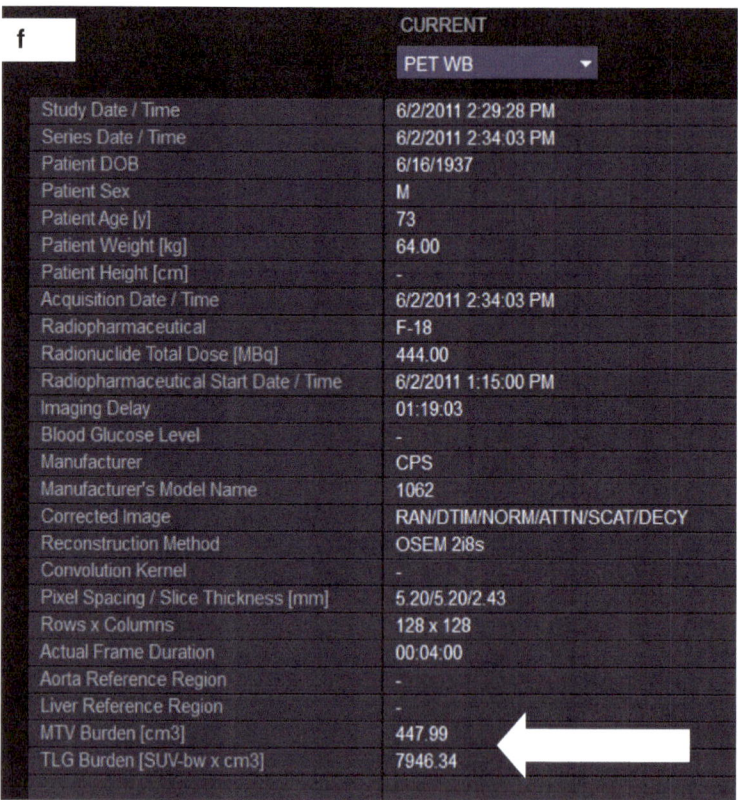

f	CURRENT
	PET WB ▼
Study Date / Time	6/2/2011 2:29:28 PM
Series Date / Time	6/2/2011 2:34:03 PM
Patient DOB	6/16/1937
Patient Sex	M
Patient Age [y]	73
Patient Weight [kg]	64.00
Patient Height [cm]	-
Acquisition Date / Time	6/2/2011 2:34:03 PM
Radiopharmaceutical	F-18
Radionuclide Total Dose [MBq]	444.00
Radiopharmaceutical Start Date / Time	6/2/2011 1:15:00 PM
Imaging Delay	01:19:03
Blood Glucose Level	-
Manufacturer	CPS
Manufacturer's Model Name	1062
Corrected Image	RAN/DTIM/NORM/ATTN/SCAT/DECY
Reconstruction Method	OSEM 2i8s
Convolution Kernel	-
Pixel Spacing / Slice Thickness [mm]	5.20/5.20/2.43
Rows x Columns	128 x 128
Actual Frame Duration	00:04:00
Aorta Reference Region	-
Liver Reference Region	-
MTV Burden [cm3]	447.99
TLG Burden [SUV-bw x cm3]	7946.34

Fig. 5.2 (continued)

5.5   Other Considerations

SUV values may vary according to different clinical and equipment parameters in ^{18}F-fluoride PET/CT. These numbers may fluctuate depending on the patient's height, weight, and bone region [15] and even different equipment with Time-of-flight (TOF) mode. Nevertheless, SUV values in ^{18}F-fluoride PET/CT are reproducible [12], have shown only modest variations in TOF mode [16], and have been validated for normal bone and for metastatic lesions and quantification can already be routinely used [17].

5.6   Conclusions

^{18}F-fluoride PET/CT volumetric quantifications play an important role as an imaging biomarker for evaluation of prognosis and response to therapy. Clinical use is validated for semi-automatic quantification.

References

1. Larson SM, Erdi Y, Akhurst T, et al. Tumor treatment response based on visual and quantitative changes in global tumor glycolysis using PET-FDG imaging. The visual response score and the change in total lesion glycolysis. Clin Positron Imaging. 1999;2: 159–71.
2. Rahim MK, Kim SE, So H, et al. Recent trends in PET image interpretations using volumetric and texture-based quantification methods in nuclear oncology. Nucl Med Mol Imaging. 2014;48:1–15.
3. Etchebehere EC, Araujo JC, Fox PS, Swanston NM, Macapinlac HA, Rohren EM. Prognostic factors in patients treated with 223Ra: the role of skeletal tumor burden on baseline ^{18}F-fluoride PET/CT in predicting overall survival. J Nucl Med. 2015;56:1177–84.
4. Etchebehere EC, Araujo JC, Milton DR, et al. Skeletal tumor burden on baseline ^{18}F-fluoride PET/CT predicts bone marrow failure after 223Ra therapy. Clin Nucl Med. 2016;41: 268–73.
5. Wassberg C, Lubberink M, Sörensen J, Johansson S. Repeatability of quantitative parameters of ^{18}F-fluoride PET/CT and biochemical tumour and specific bone remodelling markers in prostate cancer bone metastases. EJNMMI Res. 2017;7:42.
6. Brito AE, Santos A, Sasse AD, et al. ^{18}F-Fluoride PET/CT tumor burden quantification predicts survival in breast cancer. Oncotarget. 2017;8:36001.
7. Brito AET, Mourato F, Santos A, Mosci C, Ramos C, Etchebehere E. Validation of the semi-automatic quantification of ^{18}F-fluoride PET/CT whole-body skeletal tumor burden. J Nucl Med Technol. 2018;46:378.
8. Lapa P, Marques M, Costa G, Iagaru A, Pedroso de Lima J. Assessment of skeletal tumour burden on ^{18}F-NaF PET/CT using a new quantitative method. Nucl Med Commun. 2017;38:325–32.
9. Oldan J, Hawkins A, Chin B. ^{18}F sodium fluoride PET/CT in patients with prostate cancer: quantification of normal tissues, benign degenerative lesions, and malignant lesions. World J Nucl Med. 2016;15:102.

10. Sabbah N, Jackson T, Mosci C, et al. ^{18}F-sodium fluoride PET/CT in oncology. Clin Nucl Med. 2015;40:e228–31.
11. Boellaard R, Delgado-Bolton R, Oyen WJG, et al. FDG PET/CT: EANM procedure guidelines for tumour imaging: version 2.0. Eur J Nucl Med Mol Imaging. 2014;42:328–54.
12. Rohren EM, Etchebehere EC, Araujo JC, et al. Determination of skeletal tumor burden on ^{18}F-fluoride PET/CT. J Nucl Med. 2015;56:1507–12.
13. Lin C, Bradshaw T, Perk T, et al. Repeatability of quantitative ^{18}F-NaF PET: a multicenter study. J Nucl Med. 2016;57:1872–9.
14. Taghanaki SA, Duggan N, Ma H, et al. Segmentation-free direct tumor volume and metabolic activity estimation from PET scans. Comput Med Imaging Graph. 2017;63:52–66.
15. Win AZ, Aparici CM. Factors affecting uptake of NaF-18 by the normal skeleton. J Clin Med Res. 2014;6:435.
16. Oldan JD, Turkington TG, Choudhury K, Chin BB. Quantitative differences in [^{18}F] NaF PET/CT: TOF versus non-TOF measurements. Am J Nucl Med Mol Imaging. 2015;5:504–14.
17. Win AZ, Aparici CM. Normal SUV values measured from NaF18- PET/CT bone scan studies. PLoS One. 2014;9:e108429.

^18F-Fluoride: Benign Bone Disease

6

Kalevi Kairemo and Homer A. Macapinlac

Contents

6.1 Introduction

Multiple studies support the application of NaF-PET to assess benign osseous conditions. In particular, bone turnover can be measured from NaF uptake to diagnose osteoporosis. Several studies have evaluated the efficacy of bisphosphonates and their lasting effects as treatment for osteoporosis using bone turnover measured by NaF-PET [1]. Additionally, NaF uptake in vessels tracks calcification in the plaques at the molecular level, which is relevant to coronary artery disease (presented in

K. Kairemo (✉)
Department of Nuclear Medicine and Molecular Radiotherapy, Docrates Cancer Center, Helsinki, Finland

Department of Nuclear Medicine, University of Texas MD Anderson Cancer Center, Houston, TX, USA

H. A. Macapinlac
Department of Nuclear Medicine, University of Texas MD Anderson Cancer Center, Houston, TX, USA

© Springer Nature Switzerland AG 2020
K. Kairemo, H. A. Macapinlac (eds.), *Sodium Fluoride PET/CT in Clinical Use*,
Clinicians' Guides to Radionuclide Hybrid Imaging,
https://doi.org/10.1007/978-3-030-23577-2_6

Chaps. 10 and 11). Also, NaF-PET imaging of diseased joints is able to project disease progression in osteoarthritis, rheumatoid arthritis, and ankylosing spondylitis. Further studies suggest potential use of NaF-PET in domains such as back pain, osteosarcoma, stress-related fracture, and bisphosphonate-induced osteonecrosis of the jaw. The critical role of NaF-PET in disease detection and characterization of many musculoskeletal disorders has been clearly demonstrated in the literature, and these methods will become more widespread in the future. The data from PET imaging are quantitative in nature, and as such, it adds a major dimension to assessing disease activity.

NaF-PET/CT imaging (using ^{18}F-fluoride) is not a tumor-specific imaging study. The uptake of fluoride is related to multiple factors including flow and microenvironment, and as a result multiple conditions can give rise to focally increased fluoride uptake in the skeleton.

In the clinical use of NaF-PET/CT, recognition of benign conditions that may give rise to increased fluoride uptake is important so as to avoid erroneous over diagnosis of malignant conditions. Similarly, there are certain bone conditions that, although benign, are nevertheless important to recognize as they may hold clinical relevance, either as an explanation for symptoms or as a process that may prompt or guide treatment. Furthermore, with the clinical application of volumetric analytic methods such as the total fluoride index (e.g., TFI_{10}) ([2], Chap. 5) care must be taken to exclude regions of benign fluoride uptake that could interfere with the results.

In this chapter, several benign conditions that can result in increased fluoride uptake will be presented.

6.2   Normal Bone

After administration, fluoride ions localize via adsorption to the hydroxyapatite matrix of bone, and can thereby serve as a marker of bone structure and density. In fact, NaF imaging has been investigated as a means to quantitatively determine bone density, and to follow the effects of treatment for osteoporosis [3].

However, because the localization of radiotracer (both fluoride and others) is directly affected by perfusion, such studies are typically done using dynamic imaging (Chap. 7) and arterial sampling, limiting clinical utility. Nevertheless, the link between fluoride uptake and bone biology provides insight into the normal distribution of fluoride in the skeleton, whereby some bones and bone regions show higher degrees of uptake, whereas others show lower uptake. Out of 543 bone regions analyzed, the average SUV for normal skeleton fell between 3.90 and 6.62, with the majority of measurements being <10; this is the basis of the so-termed the total fluoride index TFI_{10} [2]. However, there is no automated technique that can reliably assign areas of increased fluoride uptake to physiological, benign, or malignant processes, and a physician-directed manipulation is required to accurately generate a disease specific TFI_{10}. Areas of benign uptake (as determined by the readers/clinical data) may show high SUVs as well, with significant overlap to the malignant lesions.

6.3   Arthropathic Disease

Apart from areas of normal skeletal heterogeneity related to bone structure and remodeling, perhaps the most common cause of increased fluoride uptake in the skeleton is arthropathy such as inflammatory arthritis, osteoarthritis, spondyloarthropathy, and others [1]. Typically in older patients being imaged with NaF-PET/CT for evaluation of malignancy, arthropathy, particularly degenerative disease, is a very common occurrence.

Depending on the etiology, the appearance and distribution of fluoride uptake can vary, but typically the uptake is in or adjacent to the joint spaces. Osteoarthropathy will often involve the large joints including the hips and knees, as well as the vertebral facet joints. Other joints can be involved, as well, including the shoulders, wrists, and interphalangeal joints. Nonsynovial joints and articulations may also show degenerative changes that manifest with increased fluoride uptake, most commonly the intervertebral disk spaces and vertebral end plates.

A careful review of the CT images can often confirm the presence of ancillary features confirmatory of arthropathy, such as joint space narrowing, erosions, and subchondral sclerosis.

With regard to one of the most commonly encountered sites of joint pathology, osteoarthropathy of the hip, NaF-PET/CT may provide helpful clinical information. A study of patients with this disease was performed using fluoride imaging, and among 57 hip joints analyzed, the authors found SUVmax to be highly correlated with risk for pain worsening and progression of joint space narrowing [4]. In another common disease, rheumatoid arthritis, NaF-PET/CT was found to be complimentary to metabolic imaging, with FDG-PET/CT demonstrating proliferative changes not only in the synovial soft tissues but also in the periarticular bone [5]. In this study, it was furthermore observed that patients with high NaF uptake were those with erosive disease, a feature of aggressive rheumatoid arthritis.

In the spondyloarthropathies, particular interest has been given to ankylosing spondylitis (AS) and sacroiliitis, as these conditions are challenging with regard to both diagnosis and monitoring of therapy effects. Preliminary studies have suggested a role for NaF-PET/CT imaging in these patients. In one study of 29 patients with AS, the authors found a link between NaF-PET/CT imaging findings and clinical evidence of disease using the Bath Ankylosing Spondylitis Disease Activity Index and Ankylosing Spondylitis Disease Activity Score [6]. Additionally, functional activity and disease activity in AS patients could be characterized with only a single NaF-PET/CT study.

PET/MRI with NaF may also have a role in the evaluation of patients with spondyloarthropathy. The combination of the 2 imaging techniques was proposed to provide synergistic information regarding the disease status, due to the superior tissue contrast resolution of MRI, combined with the sensitivity of fluoride PET for bone structure and turnover. Indeed, the authors of the study, in evaluating 13 patients with AS using NaF-PET/MR, found that there was benefit to the inclusion of the MR finding of bone marrow edema and fat deposition along with the intensity of fluoride uptake in the determination of disease activity in AS [7]. PET/CT data suggest that AS activity is reflected by bone activity (formation) rather than inflammation.

6.4 Bone Remodeling and Repair

Because of the link between bone metabolism and fluoride uptake, a variety of benign conditions can result in either focal or diffuse abnormalities of fluoride uptake on NaF-PET/CT imaging. The degree and intensity of activity may vary with the age of the process, the degree of perfusion, and the anatomic location and local bone structure. In some cases, benign uptake due to inflammatory or reparative processes can be mistaken for malignancy [1].

A common cause of focal bone uptake in patients undergoing NaF-PET/CT is healing fracture. The presence of uptake in healing bone has been long recognized through experience with conventional bone scintigraphy. NaF-PET/CT, with its superior sensitivity and spatial resolution, may likewise highlight (often to an even greater degree than bone scanning) areas of bone repair and callus formation. In the older population undergoing fluoride bone imaging for detection of osseous metastatic disease, it is important to recognize benign uptake because of fracture to avoid false positive interpretation. As with conventional bone scintigraphy, the pattern of uptake may sometimes offer clues as to the benign nature of the uptake. It is crucial, however, to utilize the information on CT to identify and confirm the presence of fracture, through the observation of cortical discontinuity, nonaggressive periosteal reaction, or linearly configured sclerosis. In questionable cases, e.g., plain radiography or MRI can be employed to further characterize the findings. In some cases, detection of fractures is critically important and may indeed be the rationale for performance of NaF-PET/CT. Several studies have examined the use of NaF-PET/CT in the evaluation of occult fractures in children as a sign of abuse [8].

Other causes of bone damage can also result in increased fluoride uptake. Bone infarction can occur in various settings by which the blood supply to bone is impaired or interrupted, resulting in areas of marrow or cortical necrosis followed by healing and repair.

Bone infarction is an example of a process in which various phases of disease show differential patterns of radiotracer uptake. Typically, the acute phase of bone infarction is characterized by diminished tracer accumulation because of impaired perfusion.

In the following reparative phase, tracer uptake is often increased because of matrix formation and calcification. In the later phases, tracer uptake can remain elevated, or may normalize. A variety of disorders can result in bone infarction, including trauma, hemoglobinopathy (e.g., sickle cell anemia), and corticosteroid use. As with conventional bone scintigraphy, NaF-PET/CT can provide information in patients with known or suspected osteomyelitis.

Although not routinely performed, it has been shown that dynamic NaF-PET/CT imaging is feasible (Chap. 7) to capture characteristics of hyperemia and vascular permeability, the same rationale for the performance of conventional bone scintigraphy in a dynamic (i.e., three-phase) fashion for evaluation of bone infection. Several studies have examined the potential role of fluoride PET/CT in the evaluation of suspected postoperative infection [9] and infected prostheses [10], although neither indication is in routine clinical use. It is unclear what role NaF-PET/CT imaging will have in the evaluation of infection, compared to other standard imaging techniques such as FDG-PET/CT or labeled infection homing blood cells.

6.5   Foot Pain of Unclear Cause

There has been some attempts to analyze the role of NaF-PET/CT imaging in assessing the cause of foot pain. One study compared the quality and diagnostic performance of ^{18}F-fluoride PET/MR imaging with that of ^{18}F-fluoride PET/CT imaging in 22 patients with foot pain of unclear cause [11]. The sensitivity of the PET datasets in PET/MR and PET/CT was equivalent, with the same 42 lesions showing focal ^{18}F-fluoride uptake. A final consensus interpretation revealed the most frequent main diagnoses to be osteoarthritis, stress fracture, and bone marrow edema. PET/CT was more precise in visualizing osteoarthritis, but PET/MR combined the high sensitivity of ^{18}F-fluoride PET to pinpoint areas with the dominant disease activity and the specificity of MR imaging for the final diagnosis [11].

In another study patient management was affected by findings of ^{18}F-fluoride PET/CT in 31 out of 61 painful lesions (50.8%) in 31 patients who had 16 lesions in forefoot (26.2%), 11 in midfoot (18.0%), 19 in hind foot (31.2%), 6 in ankle (9.8%), and 9 diffuse foot pain (14.8%) [12].

6.6   Benign Focal Bone Lesions

There is a wide range of histologically benign bone lesions that can either be discovered incidentally in patients undergoing imaging for other reasons, or detected intentionally because of signs or symptoms. A systematic review of these lesions is well beyond the scope of this book chapter, and books and reviews have been written detailing the incidence, pathophysiology, and imaging appearances of these lesions. Anyway, these are of importance in the differential diagnosis. Some of these conditions are listed in Table 6.1.

Table 6.1 List of benign bone lesions can be found by NaF-PET/CT	Fibrous dysplasia
	Enchondroma/eosinophilic granuloma
	Giant cell tumor of bone
	Nonossifying fibroma
	Osteoblastoma
	Metastases/myeloma (that can appear benign radiographically)
	Aneurysmal bone cyst
	Simple (or unicameral) bone cyst
	Hyperparathyroidism (brown tumors)
	Infection
	Chondroblastoma/chondromyxoid fibroma
	Paget's disease
	Melorheostosis
	Gorham-Stout disease

Extensive NaF uptake can be found, e.g., in melorheostosis and Paget disease including ossified soft tissues. Melorheostosis is a rare, nonhereditary, benign, sclerotic bone dysplasia with no sex predilection, typically occurring in late childhood or early adulthood, which can lead to substantial functional morbidity [13]. Paget's disease (PD) of bone is a benign but chronic disorder of bone metabolism. A case with several fractures in the pelvis and radiograph raising suspicion of metastases has been reported [14]. An F-NaF PET/CT demonstrated high F-NaF uptake in the same regions to the differential diagnosis with metastatic lesions.

As an example, Gorham-Stout disease (GSD) is an extremely rare skeletal disorder of unknown etiology characterized by benign proliferation of vascular or lymphatic channels, leading to progressive bone resorption. A case reported in the literature did not show F-FDG uptake but demonstrated markedly increased F-NaF activity [15].

In general, incidentally detected skeletal lesions can show varying patterns of radiotracer uptake on NaF-PET/CT. The uptake must be correlated with the radiographic characteristics, location, and patient information to determine whether a particular lesion is, indeed, because of a benign cause or related to malignancy. Again, plain radiographs can be most helpful because of their superior spatial resolution and characterization of bone structure, and MRI may be a complementary technique in difficult cases.

6.7 Conclusions

As the use of clinical NaF-PET/CT imaging becomes more widespread and available, it is unavoidable that benign causes of fluoride uptake will be encountered in day-to-day practice.

As the majority of these fluoride scans will be performed for detection or characterization of osseous metastatic disease, recognition of benign causes of fluoride uptake is critical to over diagnosis and upstaging. In cases where skeletal disease burden is quantified for purposes of prognosis, care must be taken to differentiate the areas of malignant skeletal involvement from those resulting from benign processes such as fracture repair and inflammation. Ultimately, the best interpretation of NaF-PET/CT arises from a careful review of both the PET images and the CT (or increasingly, MR) images for determination of anatomy and structure.

References

1. Rohren EM, Macapinlac HA. Spectrum of benign bone conditions on NaF-PET. Semin Nucl Med. 2017;47:392–6.
2. Rohren EM, Etchebehere EC, Araujo JC, et al. Determination of skeletal tumor burden on ^{18}F-fluoride PET/CT. J Nucl Med. 2015;56:1507–12.

3. Uchida K, Nakajima H, Miyazaki T, et al. Effects of alendronate on bone metabolism in glucocorticoid-induced osteoporosis measured by 18F-fluoride PET: a prospective study. J Nucl Med. 2009;50:1808–14.

4. Kobayashi N, Inaba Y, Yukizawa Y, et al. Use of 18F-fluoride positron emission tomography as a predictor of hip osteoarthritis progression. Mod Rheumatol. 2015;25:925–30.

5. Watanabe T, Takase-Minegishi K, Ihata A, et al. 18F-FDG and 18F-NaF PET/CT demonstrate coupling of inflammation and accelerated bone turnover in rheumatoid arthritis. Mod Rheumatol. 2016;26:180–7.

6. Idolazzi L, Salgarello M, Gatti D, et al. 18F-fluoride PET/CT for detection of axial involvement in ankylosing spondylitis: correlation with disease activity. Ann Nucl Med. 2016;30:430–4.

7. Buchbender C, Ostendorf B, Ruhlmann V, et al. Hybrid 18F-labeled fluoride positron emission tomography/magnetic resonance (MR) imaging of the sacroiliac joints and the spine in patients with axial spondyloarthritis: a pilot study exploring the link of MR bone pathologies and increased osteoblastic activity. J Rheumatol. 2015;42:1631–7.

8. Grant FD. 18F-fluoride PET and PET/CT in children and young adults. PET Clin. 2014;9:287–97.

9. Shim JJ, Lee JW, Jeon MH, et al. Recurrent surgical site infection of the spine diagnosed by dual 18F-NaF-bone PET/CT with early-phase scan. Skelet Radiol. 2016;45:1313–6.

10. Kumar R, Kumar R, Kumar V, et al. Comparative analysis of dual-phase 18F-fluoride PET/CT and three phase bone scintigraphy in the evaluation of septic (or painful) hip prostheses: a prospective study. J Orthop Sci. 2016;21:205–10.

11. Rauscher I, Beer AJ, Schaeffeler C, et al. Evaluation of 18F-fluoride PET/MR and PET/CT in patients with foot pain of unclear cause. J Nucl Med. 2015;56:430–5.

12. Kim JY, Choi YY, Kim YH, Park SB, Jeong MA. Role of (18)F-fluoride PET/CT over dual-phase bone scintigraphy in evaluation and management of lesions causing foot and ankle pain. Ann Nucl Med. 2015;29:302–12.

13. Papadakis GZ, Jha S, Bhattacharyya T, et al. 18F-NaF PET/CT in extensive melorheostosis of the axial and appendicular skeleton with soft-tissue involvement. Clin Nucl Med. 2017;42:537–9.

14. Cucchi F, Simonsen L, Abild-Nielsen AG, Broholm R. 18F-sodium fluoride PET/CT in Paget disease. Clin Nucl Med. 2017;42:553–4.

15. Papadakis GZ, Millo C, Bagci U, Blau J, Collins MT. 18F-NaF and 18F-FDG PET/CT in Gorham-Stout disease. Clin Nucl Med. 2016;41:884–5.

Dynamic ¹⁸F-Fluoride Imaging

7

Homer A. Macapinlac and Kalevi Kairemo

Contents

7.1 Introduction

Diseases affecting bone metabolism involve a wide range of skeletal and soft tissue disorders. They may be grouped as osteoporosis, osteomalacia, hyperparathyroidism, Paget's disease of bone, and developmental disorders of bone. Age-related osteoporosis alone affects about 28 million Americans, and the cost of caring for osteoporosis-related fractures has recently been estimated to be about $14.8 billion each year.

Bone metabolic biomarkers to assess osteoclastic bone resorption such as the N- or C-terminus telopeptides or osteoblastic bone formation such as alkaline

H. A. Macapinlac
Department of Nuclear Medicine, University of Texas MD Anderson Cancer Center, Houston, TX, USA

K. Kairemo (✉)
Department of Nuclear Medicine, University of Texas MD Anderson Cancer Center, Houston, TX, USA

Department of Nuclear Medicine and Molecular Radiotherapy, Docrates Cancer Center, Helsinki, Finland

© Springer Nature Switzerland AG 2020
K. Kairemo, H. A. Macapinlac (eds.), *Sodium Fluoride PET/CT in Clinical Use*,
Clinicians' Guides to Radionuclide Hybrid Imaging,
https://doi.org/10.1007/978-3-030-23577-2_7

phosphatase or procollagen type-1 N/C- propeptide and bone mineral density techniques (e.g., dual-energy X-ray absorptiometry or DXA) are used as surrogates to assess effectiveness of fracture prevention therapies. However, biomarkers do not assess specific sites and reflect changes throughout the skeleton. On the other hand, although DXA is site specific for the forearm, lumbar spine, and hips, it usually take 2 or more years to evaluate the effect of therapy on bone mass [1].

7.2   Technique and Applications

The earliest studies to interrogate bone metabolism with nuclear medicine techniques utilized ^{99m}Tc-MDP first with whole body counting, and later with gamma camera imaging and blood sampling. Dynamic NaF PET allows the quantitative assessment of bone formation by measuring the clearance of fluoride to bone in any region imaged. The Hawkins method ushered in the use of PET imaging utilizing ^{18}F NaF which required a 60-min dynamic acquisition, CT for attenuation correction and measurement of arterial input function with either direct arterial sampling or image derived input from the aorta/femoral artery or venous sampling [2]. Although arterial sampling may provide the most robust data, simpler venous sampling techniques utilizing a semi-population input function have been done and may serve as an alternative technique [3]. Nevertheless, the arterial input function needs to be combined with the bone time activity curves on the dynamic PET scan to derive the plasma clearance of each region of interest. Analysis is done using the Hawkins compartmental model (Fig. 7.1) to allow calculation of parameter Ki which represents net plasma clearance (see Fig. 7.1).

$$\left(K_i = K_1 \times k_3 \, / \left(k_2 + k_3 \right) \mathrm{ml\,min^{-1}\,ml^{-1}} \right). \tag{7.1}$$

Patlak quantitative analysis can be done as a graphical method of measuring K_i assuming that k_4 is small and negligible. A modified Holden technique was applied by Siddique method to measure PET scans of the spine and hip [4].

A simplified method of static PET image acquisition and analysis was proposed by Siddique [4], Table 7.1 demonstrates the method. This requires static imaging over the lumbar spine and hips at 45–60 min post injection and a semi-population input function with venous sampling taken at baseline and 30 min post injection. The simplified method may potentially be more acceptable to patients (shorter camera time) and does not require an arterial stick. What is needed are more clinical studies utilizing this technique to assess responders and nonresponders to new treatments for osteoporosis [1].

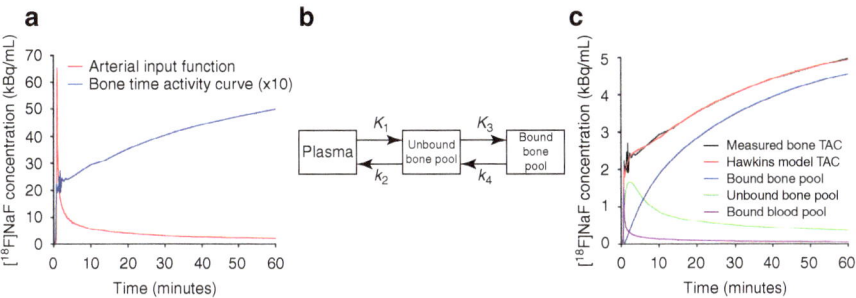

Fig. 7.1 Quantitative analysis using the Hawkins model. (**a**) Representative curves showing the arterial input function measured by direct blood sampling and corresponding bone time activity curve (TAC) for a [¹⁸F]NaF dynamic PET scan of the lumbar spine. Both curves have been corrected for radioactive decay. Reproduced with permission from [1]. (**b**) The Hawkins compartmental model used for the analysis of [¹⁸F]NaF PET dynamic bone scans. The rate constant K_1 describes the effective bone plasma flow to the unbound bone pool, k_2 the reverse transport of tracer from the unbound bone pool back to plasma, k_3 the forward transport from the unbound bone pool to bone mineral, and k_4 the reverse flow. Bone plasma clearance K_i is calculated using Eq. (7.1). (**c**) Results of fitting the bone TAC and arterial plasma input function to the Hawkins compartmental model. In addition to the 4 parameters K_1, k_2, k_3, and k_4 the model also fits the fractional volume of blood within the bone ROI, FBV. The plasma clearance to bone mineral K_i is calculated using Eq. (7.1). The figure shows time activity plots of the amount of tracer in each compartment of the Hawkins model and the resulting fit of the summed curves to the measured bone TAC. [¹⁸F]NaF, fluorine-18 labelled sodium fluoride; *PET* positron emission tomography

Table 7.1   Protocol for dynamic NaF PET using static scanning (modified from [4])

Simplified protocol for [¹⁸F]NaF PET imaging using static scan method
Injected activity: 90 MBq (spine) or 180 MBq (hip) [¹⁸F]NaF in 10 ml saline
Acquisition of static scan sequence commences at 45–60 min and should be completed by 75–80 min
Patient should empty their bladder before scanning
CT scan and 5-min static PET scan at each measurement site
Positioning: spine: L1–L4 including bottom of Th12 and top of L5
Hip: 1 cm above acetabulum to mid-femoral shaft
Other sites: Up to whole body, if required
Measurement of arterial input function: semi-population input function with venous samples taken at 30 min after injection, before the start and after completing the static scan sequence

[¹⁸F]NaF fluorine-18 labelled sodium fluoride, *PET* positron emission tomography

7.3   Tumor Imaging

Dynamic PET imaging was applied by Sachpekidis et al. to 80 multiple myeloma (MM) patients undergoing high dose chemotherapy and autologous stem cell transplantation to distinguish benign from malignant lesions; 263 myeloma lesions were demonstrated. Semi-quantitative and quantitative evaluations were performed for 25 MM lesions as well as for 25 benign, degenerative, and traumatic lesions. Unfortunately, no statistically significant differences between MM and benign degenerative disease regarding $SUV_{average}$, SUV_{max}, K_1, k_3, and influx (K_i) were demonstrated [5]. Interestingly, the same group compared NaF and FDG PET/CT in 29 multiple myeloma patients to assess response. Although FDG had limited sensitivity, it seemed suitable for response assessment, and NaF did not add significantly to treatment response evaluation [6].

A pilot study of 6 patients by Simoncic et al. compared dynamic FDG and NaF PET/CT scanning in sequential fashion in patients with metastatic prostate cancer undergoing therapy with ZA4054. Baseline scans 4 weeks on the drug and week six after a drug break were performed. The study concluded that late NaF and FDG uptake responses are consistently correlated but that earlier uptake responses and all vasculature responses can be unrelated [7].

7.4   Non-tumor Imaging Applications

Multiple non-oncologic applications outside of osteoporosis have been done in the subspeciality of orthopedics. A pilot study in 6 patients with facetogenic low back pain was performed with dynamic NaF PET/MR imaging, to correlate clinical measures of disability with dynamic PET metrics, MR grading of lumbar facet arthropathy. The authors suggest that dynamic NaF PET may be a useful biomarker for facetogenic disability as it had a significant correlation between maximum fact joint uptake rate and clinical disability [8]. Joint replacements can fail due to infections, dislocation, fracture, or loosening. But distinguishing infection from aseptic loosening is important as the management is different. A review of the role of dynamic NaF PET imaging was done to assess its role in distinguishing septic from aseptic failure in hip and knee joint replacements. They found 3 prospective studies and the sensitivity of NaF PET in identifying prosthesis infections was found to be 97.0%, calculated from the weighted average sensitivity from the three different studies. The weighted specificity, PPV, NPV, and accuracy are 88.1, 84.7, 98.8, and 87.3%, respectively [9]. They concluded that aside from being sensitive and specific, the addition of the CT component further enhances its diagnostic and interventional radiology value.

A pilot study utilizing dynamic NaF PET was performed in 11 patients to assess feasibility of the early phases of tracer distribution in patients with chronic osteomyelitis. The findings were similar to that of a 3 phase bone scan and could potentially lead to comparative trials with Tc-99m MDP [10].

In conclusion dynamic NaF PET/CT is a promising technique which has complemented standard bone turnover measurements such as biochemical markers and bone densitometry studies. The dynamic PET technique with the advent of hybrid PET/CT imaging machines with refinements in image acquisition may make it more clinically feasible (faster imaging) with less invasive needs for blood drawing (venous versus arterial). It may provide a method to assess response to treatments for osteoporosis, various tumor types, and orthopedic applications.

References

1. Blake GM, Puri T, Siddique M, Frost ML, Moore AEB, Fogelman I. Site specific measurements of bone formation using [¹⁸F] sodium fluoride PET/CT. Quant Imaging Med Surg. 2018;8(1):47–59. https://doi.org/10.21037/qims.2018.01.02.
2. Hawkins RA, Choi Y, Huang SC, Hoh CK, Dahlbom M, Schiepers C, Satyamurthy N, Barrio JR, Phelps ME. Evaluation of the skeletal kinetics of fluorine-18-fluoride ion with PET. J Nucl Med. 1992;33:633–42.
3. Blake GM, Siddique M, Puri T, Frost ML, Moore AE, Cook GJ, Fogelman I. A semipopulation input function for quantifying static and dynamic ¹⁸F-fluoride PET scans. Nucl Med Commun. 2012;33:881–8.
4. Siddique M, Frost ML, Moore AE, Fogelman I, Blake GM. Correcting ¹⁸F-fluoride PET static scan measurements of skeletal plasma clearance for tracer efflux from bone. Nucl Med Commun. 2014;35:303–10.
5. Sachpekidis C, Hillengass J, Goldschmidt H, Anwar H, Haberkorn U, Dimitrakopoulou-Strauss A. Quantitative analysis of ¹⁸F-NaF dynamic PET/CT cannot differentiate malignant from benign lesions in multiple myeloma. Am J Nucl Med Mol Imaging. 2017;7(4):148–56.
6. Sachpekidis C, Hillengass J, Goldschmidt H3, Wagner B, Haberkorn U, Kopka K, Dimitrakopoulou-Strauss A. Treatment response evaluation with ¹⁸F-FDG PET/CT and ¹⁸F-NaF PET/CT in multiple myeloma patients undergoing high-dose chemotherapy and autologous stem cell transplantation. Eur J Nucl Med Mol Imaging. 2017;44(1):50–62.
7. Simoncic U, Perlman S, Liu G, Staab MJ, Straus JE, Jeraj R. Comparison of NaF and FDG PET/CT for assessment of treatment response in castration-resistant prostate cancers with osseous metastases. Clin Genitourin Cancer. 2015;13(1):e7–e17. https://doi.org/10.1016/j.clgc.2014.07.001.
8. Jenkins NW, Talbott JF, Shah V, Pandit P, Seo Y, Dillon WP, Majumdar S. [¹⁸F]-sodium fluoride PET MR-based localization and quantification of bone turnover as a biomarker for facet joint-induced disability. AJNR Am J Neuroradiol. 2017;38(10):2028–31. https://doi.org/10.3174/ajnr.A5348.
9. Adesanya O, Sprowson A, Masters J, Hutchinson C. Review of the role of dynamic ¹⁸F-NaF PET in diagnosing and distinguishing between septic and aseptic loosening in hip prosthesis. J Orthop Surg Res. 2015;10:5. https://doi.org/10.1186/s13018-014-0147-7.
10. Freesmeyer M, Stecker FF, Schierz JH, Hofmann GO, Winkens T. First experience with early dynamic ⁽¹⁸⁾F-NaF-PET/CT in patients with chronic osteomyelitis. Ann Nucl Med. 2014;28(4):314–21. https://doi.org/10.1007/s12149-014-0810-4.

[18]F-Fluoride Imaging: Atlas of Interesting Images (Images with Specific Teaching Points, Tracer, Technique, and Pitfalls)

8

Guofan Xu

Contents

8.1 Benign Bone Findings

Uptake of ^{18}F-NaF is not tumor specific, and nonmalignant entities can demonstrate radiotracer uptake, including arthritis, trauma, and bone processes such as fibrous dysplasia and Paget disease. The degree of radiotracer uptake cannot be used to differentiate benign from malignant lesions. Many benign bone lesions, including osteophytes and degenerative endplate changes, will show increased ^{18}F-NaF uptake [1].

G. Xu (✉)
Department of Nuclear Medicine, University of Texas MD Anderson Cancer Center, Houston, TX, USA
e-mail: GXu2@mdanderson.org

© Springer Nature Switzerland AG 2020   61
K. Kairemo, H. A. Macapinlac (eds.), *Sodium Fluoride PET/CT in Clinical Use*,
Clinicians' Guides to Radionuclide Hybrid Imaging,
https://doi.org/10.1007/978-3-030-23577-2_8

8.1.1   Fibrous Dysplasia

Nonmalignant uptake was caused by fibrous dysplasia in a 68-year-old woman. Axial ^{18}F-NaF PET image shows focal marked uptake (arrow) in the occipital bone. Axial CT and fused PET/CT images show an expansile ground-glass lesion with well-defined margins. This lesion is stable on a follow-up NaF PET image 1 year later, most compatible with fibrous dysplasia.

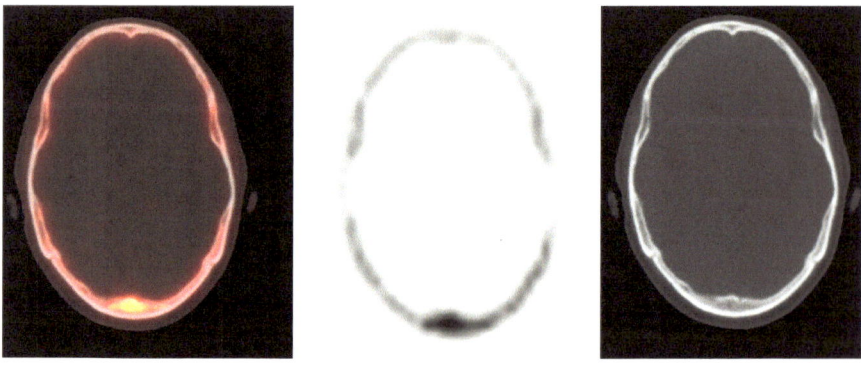

8.1.2   Shoulder Arthritis

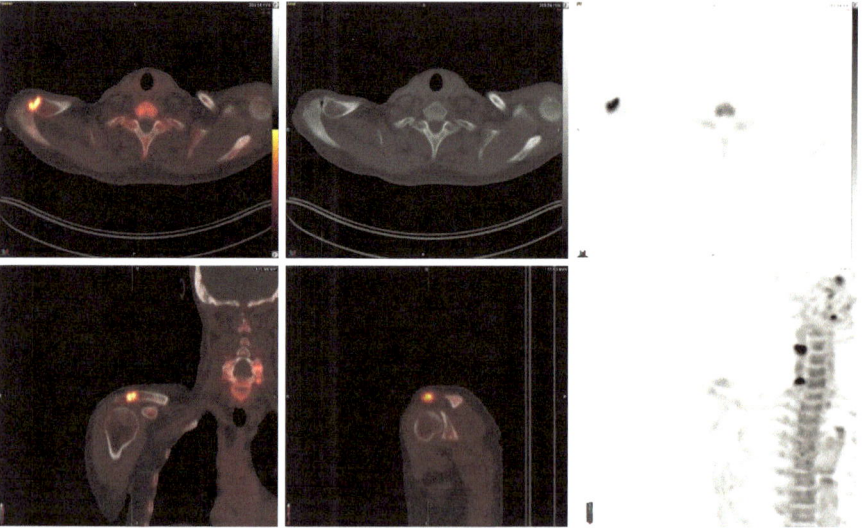

There is focal intense NaF uptake in the right shoulder acromioclavicular joint, seen on fused PET/CT and PET images. On the CT image, no aggressive osseous change is seen.

8.1.3   Rheumatoid Arthritis

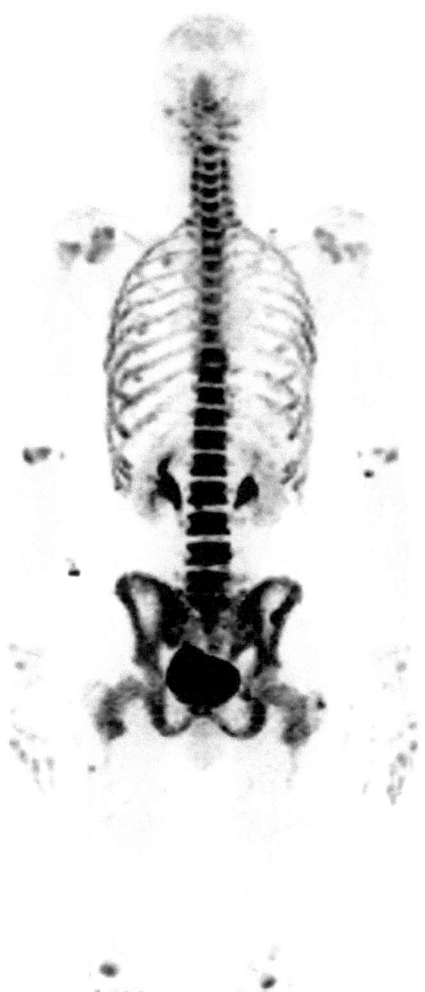

A 61-year-old woman with history of breast cancer and rhumatoid arthritis who underwent the ^{18}F-NaF PET/CT exam for cancer restaging. ^{18}F-NaF PET MIP image shows focal increased radiotracer accumulation in the shoulders, elbows, wrists, and multiple MP joints, which was related to regional hyperemia due to underlying inflammation from rheumatoid arthritis. ^{18}F-NaF PET MIP image shows increased accumulation of ^{18}F-NaF (arrows) in the shoulders, elbows, wrists, and multiple MP joints that was related to underlying rheumatoid arthritis.

Degenerative changes at MTP joint of the foot:

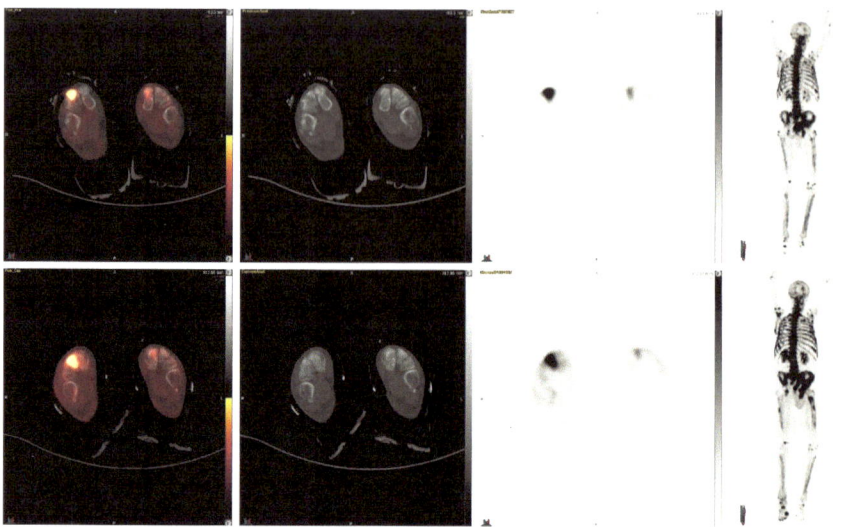

Pars fractures at L5/S1 mimicking metastatic disease

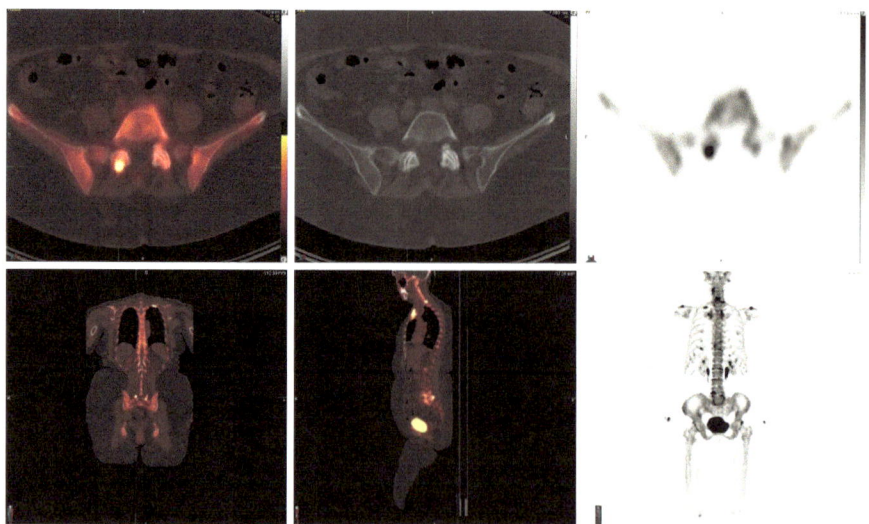

8.1.4   Traumatic Changes Mimicking Osseous Metastatic Disease

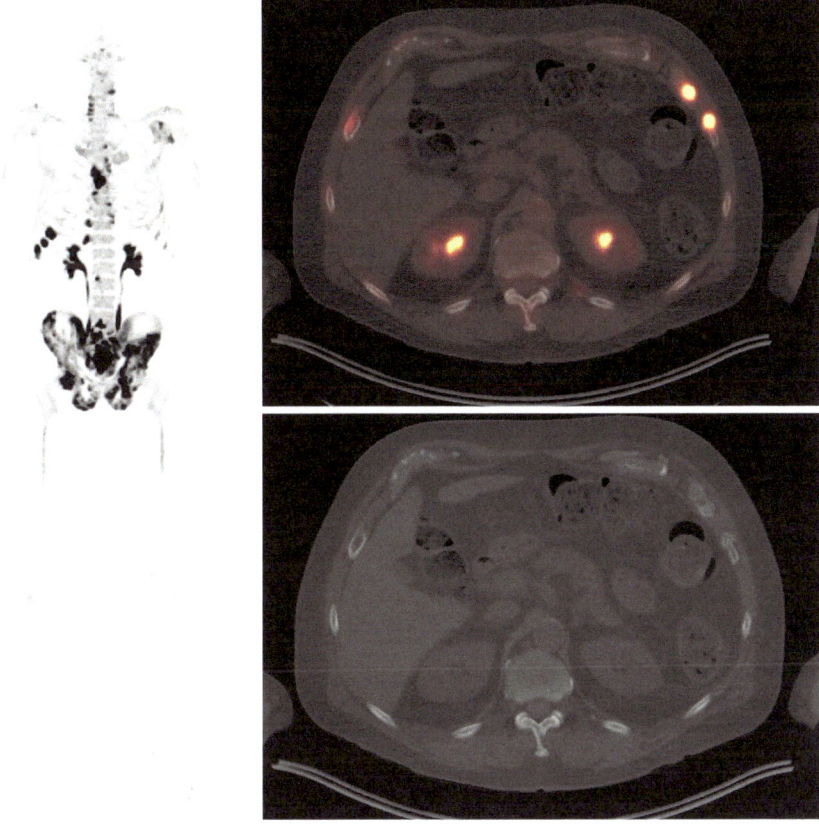

A 68-year-old male with metastatic prostate cancer who has multiple foci of avid NaF uptake in anterior left lower ribs. These foci correlate with rib fractures seen on the CT. The patient had a recent fall.

8.1.5   Urine Collection Bag

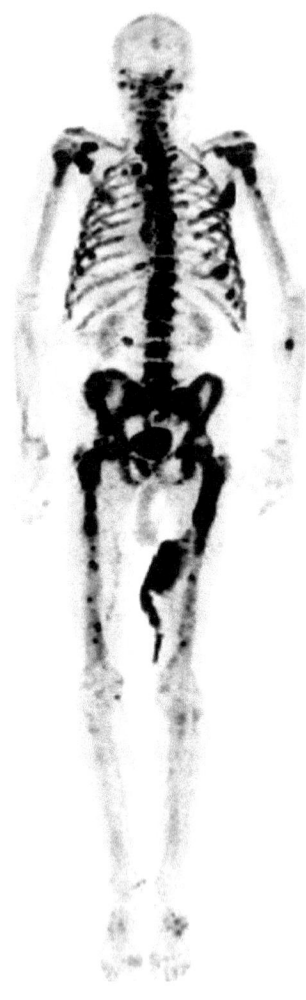

A 72-year-old male with metastatic prostate cancer. There is prominent collection of radiotracer uptake along the medial left thigh on the PET images.

8.2   Multiple Osseous Metastatic Disease

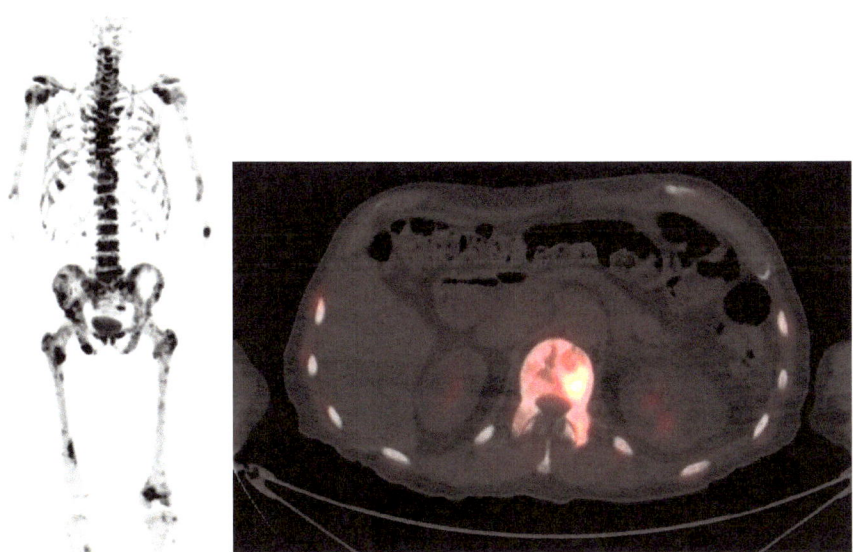

In a 62-year-old male with metastatic prostate cancer, heterogeneously avid ^{18}F-NaF uptake is seen within the axial and proximal appendicular skeleton.

Skull metastatic disease instead of sinus uptake

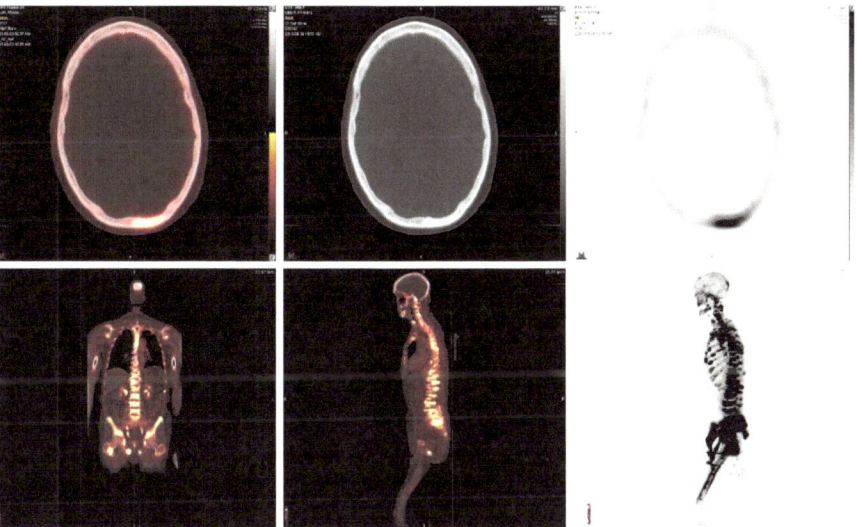

8.3   SuperScan Pattern of Metastatic Disease

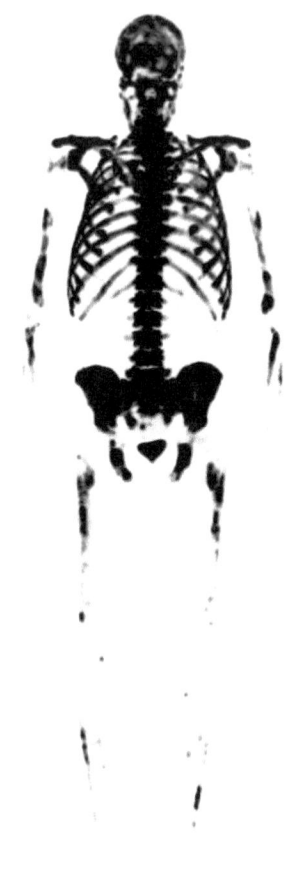

Symmetrically intense and diffuse radiotracer uptake in the skeleton with absent or diminished visualization of the genitourinary system and soft tissues.

Reference

1. Segall G, et al. SNM practice guideline for sodium ^{18}F-Fluride PET/CT bone scan 1.0. J Nucl Med. 2010;51(11):1813–20.

Role of Sodium Fluoride-PET in Primary Bone Tumors

9

Vivek Subbiah and Kalevi Kairemo

Contents

V. Subbiah

Department of Investigational Cancer Therapeutics (Phase I Clinical Trials Program), Unit 455, Division of Cancer Medicine, The University of Texas MD Anderson Cancer Center, Houston, TX, USA
e-mail: vsubbiah@mdanderson.org

K. Kairemo (✉)
Department of Nuclear Medicine and Molecular Radiotherapy, Docrates Cancer Center, Helsinki, Finland

Department of Nuclear Medicine, University of Texas MD Anderson Cancer Center, Houston, TX, USA

© Springer Nature Switzerland AG 2020
K. Kairemo, H. A. Macapinlac (eds.), *Sodium Fluoride PET/CT in Clinical Use*, Clinicians' Guides to Radionuclide Hybrid Imaging,
https://doi.org/10.1007/978-3-030-23577-2_9

9.1   Primary Bone Tumors

Malignant bone tumors are classified based on the histological origin. The nomenclature is based on the predominant components of the malignancy. Osteogenic sarcoma (osteosarcoma), chondrosarcoma, and Ewing's sarcoma are primary bone tumors. Although multiple myeloma is the most common primary bone tumor it is considered a marrow cell tumor and not one arising from the bone. The incidence of the primary bone tumors vary depending upon the age (Table 9.1). Owing to the ability to metastasize and progress rapidly they are a cause of major morbidity and mortality. Osteosarcoma and Ewing's sarcoma strike adolescents and young adults in the prime of their lives. Conventional imaging modalities for staging and restaging include bone scintigraphy with SPECT/CT, CT scan, MRI, and PET/CT scan. More recently sodium fluoride PET/CT scan has become available. The benefit of using sodium fluoride PET/CT in malignant primary bone tumors is characterized by detectable bone formation in soft-tissue. Herein, we discuss the role of sodium fluoride PET/CT scan in imaging of primary bone tumors specifically osteosarcoma and giant cell tumor of the bone. We also present the role of sodium fluoride PET/CT in staging, monitoring, and evaluation of response in malignant primary bone tumors.

9.2   Classification of Bone Tumors

Primary bone tumors can be classified based on the type of tumor and tissue of origin and can be benign or malignant. The major ones that cause morbidity are osteosarcoma and Ewing's sarcoma. (Table 9.1) shows the broad classification. Osteosarcoma has several different histopathologic variants, and all of them are characterized by formation of bone as follows: (1) conventional that include osteoblastic, chondroblastic, and fibroblastic; (2) telangiectatic; (3) small cell; (4) low grade central; (5)

Table 9.1 Characterization of primary bone tumors

Tumor origin or cell of origin	Benign	Malignant
Osteogenic	Osteoblastoma Osteoid osteoma	Osteosarcoma
Giant cell	Giant cell tumor	Malignant transformation of giant cell tumor
Chondrogenic	Osteochondroma Chondromyxoid fibroma Chondroblastoma	Chondrosarcoma
Notochord		Chordoma
Ewing's sarcoma		Ewing's sarcoma and primitive neuroectodermal tumors
Fibrous tissue	Fibroma Fibromatosis Desmoplastic fibroma	Fibrosarcoma
Other		Adamantinoma

periosteal; (6) paraosteal; (7) secondary osteosarcoma; (8) high grade surface; (9) extra-skeletal; (10) osteosarcomatous transformation of giant cell tumor of bone.

9.3 Sodium Fluoride Imaging in Bone Sarcomas

Morphologic imaging modalities such as computed tomography (CT) and magnetic resonance imaging (MRI) are all commonly used to assess osteosarcoma. In addition, fluorine-18-fluorodeoxyglucose positron emission tomography (^{18}F-FDG PET) can be used to quantify the physiologic activity of osteosarcomas, which are characterized by increased glucose uptake that leads to biochemical changes before anatomic changes [1]. Recently molecular imaging with ^{99m}Tc-MDP scintigraphy, ^{18}F-FDG PET/CT, or Na^{18}F PET/CT was used to characterize the disease in a trial of ^{223}Radium. Herein we discuss some of the cases in detail and also review the literature for current evidence.

9.4 Case 1

9.4.1 Brain Mets Case

A 29-year-old male with a history of osteosarcoma after primary chemotherapy and surgery was on surveillance [2]. At recurrence restaging scans revealed recurrence in the left ischium, right lung metastases, and metastases to the brain, specifically the cerebellum metastases. The patient received Xofigo® ^{223}RaCl$_2$ as part of the osteosarcoma radium clinical trial. Baseline scans included a positron emission tomography–computed tomography (PET/CT) bone scan using fluoride 18 (^{18}F)

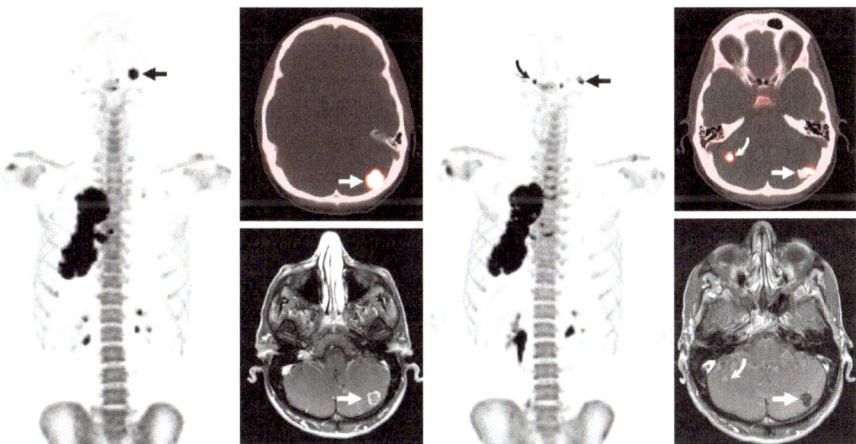

Fig. 9.1 Imaging of osteosarcoma and brain metastases and response using sodium fluoride. The responses in the brain are visualized in the bone scan and are compared with MRI of brain

(Na[18]F-PET/CT) and brain magnetic resonance imaging (MRI). After [223]RaCl$_2$ infusion with a total administered dose of 14.44 MBq (0.390 mCi) he showed a response in multiple sites including the left cerebellar metastasis. On MRI, the cerebellar lesion decreased from 1.5 cm at baseline to 1.2 cm after treatment, with resolution of perilesional edema. This was the first report of an alpha particle penetrating the blood–brain barrier and a response in the brain of a calcified sarcoma evaluated using sodium fluoride scan [2] (Fig. 9.1).

9.5   Case 2

A 54-year-old woman was diagnosed with giant cell tumor of the bone. Following several surgical resections and systemic therapy that included chemotherapy and later RANK-L inhibitor denosumab she underwent several scans as a part of staging evaluation. Patient had conventional bine scans, FDG PET/CT scans, and sodium fluoride PET scans (Fig. 9.2). More lesions quantitatively and qualitatively were visualized by sodium fluoride PET/CT scans.

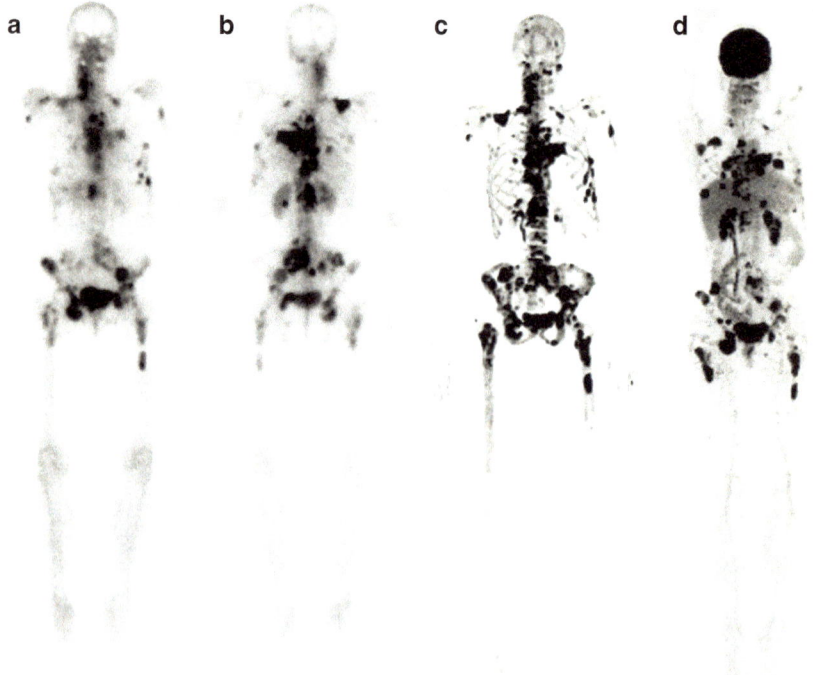

Fig. 9.2 Whole body molecular imaging studies with different techniques. Bone scintigraphy with whole-body planar images (**a**) AP-view, (**b**) P/A view, (**c**) Na[18]F-PET maximum intensity projection (MIP) images, and (**d**) [18]FDG-PET MIP images. The figure indicates that Na[18]F-PET (**c**) shows more lesions than does bone scintigraphy (**a**, **b**) (Copyright permission from BMJ Case Reports) [3]

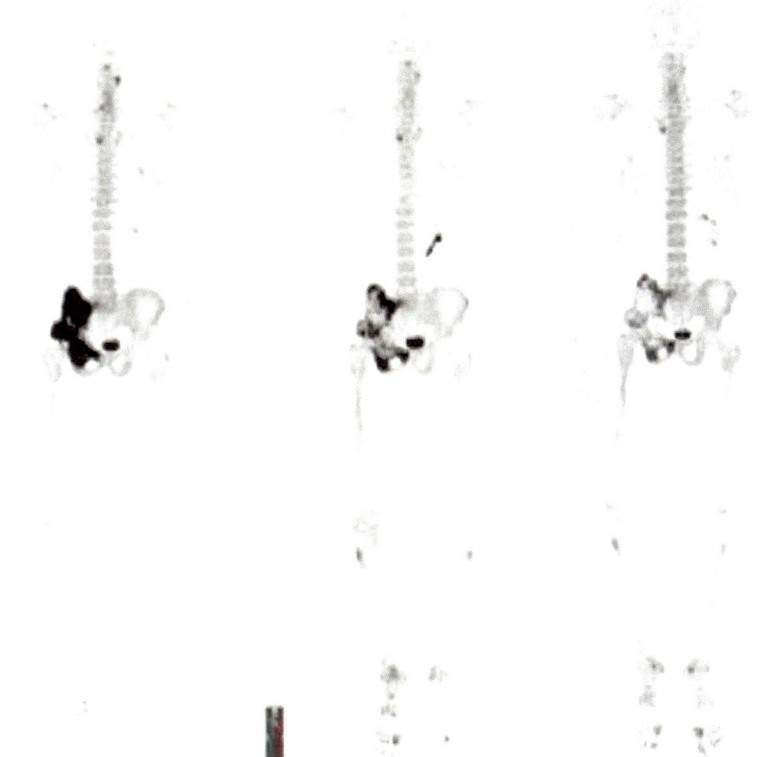

Fig. 9.3 Serial sodium fluoride-18 (Na^{18}F) images from a patient with fibroblastic osteosarcoma to the pelvis. Serial Na^{18}F positron emission tomography images at baseline, after 3 cycles of ^{223}RaCl$_2$, and after 6 cycles of ^{223}RaCl$_2$ (maximum-intensity projections). The response in the pelvic bones predominantly on the right was better visualized by Na^{18}F (Copyright permission from BMJ ESMO Open) [4]

9.6   Case 3

A male in his 60s was diagnosed with fibroblastic osteosarcoma. After several lines of chemotherapy for metastatic disease and targeted therapy he presented with pelvic pain. Because of progression he was enrolled in a clinical trial of radium-223. As part of the study he underwent sodium fluoride PET/CT scans and was noted to have significant uptake in the pelvis. After 3 doses of radium-223 he had palliation of pain and a response which could be visualized and better appreciated by sodium fluoride PET/CT scan (Fig. 9.3). After 3 more doses he had further response again visualized by sodium fluoride PET/CT scan. These subtle changes are difficult to be picked up by conventional scans like CT scan or MRI.

9.7 Review of Literature

We reviewed the literature for role of sodium fluoride in primary bone tumors. There was one case of unusual Finding of a Tumor Thrombus Arising From Osteosarcoma Detected on ^{18}F-NaF PET/CT [5] and another case of ^{18}F-NaF PET/CT unexpectedly detecting 2 foci of soft tissue increased tracer uptake in the right lateral abdominal and left paraspinal muscles, which corresponded to the focal calcification in the muscles [6]. The pathological examination revealed metastatic osteosarcoma to the muscles [6]. Combined evaluation of ^{18}F-NaF and ^{18}F-FDG PET/CT in the Evaluation of Sarcoma Patients also showed that combined F-NaF/F-FDG PET/CT scan allows for accurate evaluation of sarcoma patients [7].

9.8 Response Evaluation Using Sodium Fluoride Scans

9.8.1 Na[18]F PET Response Criteria in Solid Tumors: NAFCIST Criteria

The current Response Evaluation Criteria in Solid Tumors (RECIST) are suboptimal for use in osteosarcoma because even responding tumors do not shrink. Response in osteosarcoma neoadjuvant therapy is instead evaluated by tumor necrosis from the resected specimens. Since fluoride is taken up avidly by the bone, Na[18]F-PET/CT scan can better image the qualitative bone response to a bone targeted alpha particle therapy with Radium-223. Development of osteosarcoma therapeutics has been challenging, in part because of the lack of appropriate criteria to evaluate responses. We have shown the qualitative and quantitative approaches to metabolic tumor response assessment with Na[18]F and ^{18}F-FDG PET. We have developed a framework for Na[18]F PET response Criteria in Solid Tumors (NAFCIST), a new way to evaluate treatment response in osteosarcoma [4]. NAFCIST may be a promising criteria for high-risk osteosarcoma response evaluation [4].

In PERCIST, qualitative and quantitative approaches are used to assess the response of metabolic tumors using ^{18}F-FDG PET, with a draft framework for using RECIST with PET [1]. The MD Anderson criteria were developed as a practical approach for diagnosis and assessment of bone metastasis [8]. Response is divided into four standard categories (complete response, partial response, stable disease, and progressive disease), and the criteria include quantitative and qualitative assessments of the behavior of bone metastases. "NAFCIST" criteria takes into account the bone avid lesions in osteosarcoma. In NAFCIST, the primary outcome was determined by measuring the single most active lesion on each scan (not necessarily the same lesion). The secondary outcome was the summed activity of up to the five most intense lesions (no more than two lesions per organ) (Table 9.2).

Table 9.2 Sodium fluoride-18 (Na[18]F) Positron Emission Tomography Response Criteria in Primary Bone Tumors (NAFCIST)[a]

Response category	Criteria
Complete metabolic response	Normalization of all lesions (target and nontarget) to SUV less than mean skeletal SUV and equal to normal surrounding tissue SUV; verification with follow-up study in 1 month if anatomic criteria indicate disease progression
Partial metabolic response	>30% decrease in SUV peak[a]; verification with follow-up study if anatomic criteria indicate disease progression
Progressive metabolic disease	>30% increase in SUV peak[a]; >75% increase in total Na[18]F burden of the five most active lesions; visible increase in extent of Na[18]F uptake; new lesions; verification with follow-up study if anatomic criteria indicate complete or partial response
Stable metabolic disease	Does not meet other criteria

SUV standardized uptake value

[a]Primary outcome determination is measured on the single most active lesion on each scan (not necessarily the same lesion). Secondary outcome determination is the summed activity of up to the five most intense lesions (no more than two lesions per organ)

NAFCIST could supplant PET/CT functional response by adding metabolic response criteria for bone-forming disease. NAFCIST may represent a more accurate method of categorizing osteosarcoma than RECIST, which mainly relies on unidimensional measurements of tumor lesions and the sum of diameters.

In summary, ^{18}F-NaF PET/CT suits for osteosarcoma diagnostics not just because of its sensitivity in bone lesions, but because of possibility to analyze soft-tissue metastases due to bone formation. We also have developed new criteria (NAFCIST) for staging the disease, for disease monitoring, and quantitative evaluation of response.

Acknowledgment Funding was provided by the Shannon Wilkes osteosarcoma research program, the High-impact Clinical Research Support Program (HI-CRSP) at The University of Texas MD Anderson Cancer Center, and the National Institutes of Health Cancer Center Support Grant CA016672. The authors acknowledge Bayer for providing the radioactive isotopes.

Conflicts of Interest The funders had no role in the design and conduct of the study; collection, management, analysis, and interpretation of the data; preparation, review, or approval of the manuscript; and decision to submit the manuscript for publication.

References

1. Wahl RL, Jacene H, Kasamon Y, Lodge MA. From RECIST to PERCIST: evolving considerations for PET response criteria in solid tumors. J Nucl Med. 2009;50(Suppl 1):122S–50S.

2. Subbiah V, Anderson P, Rohren E. Alpha emitter radium 223 in high-risk osteosarcoma: first clinical evidence of response and blood-brain barrier penetration. JAMA Oncol. 2015;1(2):253–5.
3. Kairemo K, Wang WL, Subbiah V. Comprehensive molecular imaging of malignant transformation of giant cell tumor of bone reveals diverse disease biology. BMJ Case Rep. 2019;12(4). pii: e218839. https://doi.org/10.1136/bcr-2016-218839.
4. Kairemo K, Rohren EM, Anderson P, Ravizzini G, Rao A, Macapinlac HA, Subbiah V. Development of Sodium Fluoride-PET Response Criteria for Solid tumors (NAFCIST) in a clinical trial of Radium 223 in Osteosarcoma: From RECIST to PERCIST to NAFCIST. ESMO Open. 2019;4(1):e000439.
5. Verma P, Purandare N, Agrawal A, Shah S, Rangarajan V. Unusual finding of a tumor Thrombus arising from osteosarcoma detected on ^{18}F-NaF PET/CT. Clin Nucl Med. 2016;41(6):e304–6.
6. Usmani S, Marafi F, Rasheed R, Bakiratharajan D, Al Maraghy M, Al Kandari F. Unsuspected metastases to muscles in osteosarcoma detected on ^{18}F-sodium fluoride PET/CT. Clin Nucl Med. 2018;43(9):e343–e5.
7. Jackson T, Mosci C, von Eyben R, Mittra E, Ganjoo K, Biswal S, et al. Combined ^{18}F-NaF and ^{18}F-FDG PET/CT in the evaluation of sarcoma patients. Clin Nucl Med. 2015;40(9):720–4.
8. Hamaoka T, Costelloe CM, Madewell JE, Liu P, Berry DA, Islam R, et al. Tumour response interpretation with new tumour response criteria vs the World Health Organisation criteria in patients with bone-only metastatic breast cancer. Br J Cancer. 2010;102(4):651–7.

¹⁸F-Sodium Fluoride Positron Emission Tomography in Cardiac Disease

10

Marwa Daghem and David E. Newby

Contents

10.1 Introduction

Despite the recent advances, cardiovascular disease remains the leading cause of death worldwide. There is a need to improve targeting of existing novel diagnostic investigations. In the last few years, we have seen a rise in the availability of dedicated combined cardiac positron emission tomography scanners which combine molecular information from positron emission tomography with the fine anatomic detail provided by computed tomography or magnetic resonance imaging, which has in turn triggered a growing interest in the development of novel tracers providing new insight into biological disease processes. ¹⁸F-Sodium fluoride is a marker of active inflammation and calcification, and has shown promise as a novel radiotracer in cardiac imaging, having been applied in the assessment of a range of cardiac pathologies including atherosclerosis, valvular disease and cardiomyopathy.

M. Daghem (✉) · D. E. Newby
British Heart Foundation/University of Edinburgh University Centre for Cardiovascular Science, University of Edinburgh, Edinburgh, UK
e-mail: mdaghem@ed.ac.uk

© Springer Nature Switzerland AG 2020
K. Kairemo, H. A. Macapinlac (eds.), *Sodium Fluoride PET/CT in Clinical Use*,
Clinicians' Guides to Radionuclide Hybrid Imaging,
https://doi.org/10.1007/978-3-030-23577-2_10

10.2   Coronary Atherosclerosis

Atherosclerosis is an inflammatory process that affects the arterial intima with deposits of foam cells and migration of vascular smooth muscle cells. The resulting plaque causes progressive luminal stenosis and potential vessel occlusion. Calcification plays an important role in the pathogenesis of atherosclerosis. Initial calcification is thought to result from apoptosis of smooth muscle cells with the formation of micro-deposits of calcium (smaller than 50 µm), of which hydroxyapatite is the main component. It is postulated that microcalcification represents the early stages of the process and occurs as part of the healing process to intense inflammation within the necrotic core of the atheromatous plaque. In contrast, macrocalcification represents the end stages of disease with the formation of sheet-like calcification which effectively walls off the inflamed necrotic core, and stabilizes the plaque by serving as a barrier to inflammation and rupture.

The presence of calcium has long been seen as a surrogate marker of atherosclerosis and is a well-established predictor of cardiac risk [1]. Traditional computed tomography calcium scoring measures macroscopic calcification in the coronary arteries, which represents the stable stage of coronary disease. ^{18}F-Sodium fluoride can differentiate between patients with active coronary calcification which are more likely to have clinically significant coronary artery disease and a higher incidence of adverse events than those with inactive coronary macrocalcification denoting stable disease [2].

^{18}F-Sodium fluoride used in positron emission tomography imaging preferentially binds to pathological mineralization and identifies areas of microcalcification because the increased surface area of microcalcification relative to macrocalcification results in increased tracer uptake. Recent evidence demonstrates an inverse correlation between plaque calcium density and tracer uptake, with lesions at the lower end of the Hounsfield unit coefficient exhibiting greater radioisotope accumulation whilst denser and more computed tomography-evident plaque—with high calcium scores—had relatively lower fluoride uptake [3]. Moreover, ^{18}F-sodium fluoride atherosclerotic plaque uptake is related to the burden of CV risk factors but does not appear to be associated with coronary calcium score [4]. This suggests that computed tomography evidence of calcification and positron emission tomography evidence of ^{18}F-sodium fluoride uptake represent 2 different markers of atherosclerosis. The former is a surrogate marker of total plaque burden whilst the later may represent an active disease process and denote increased vulnerability [5].

Following acute myocardial infarction, increased ^{18}F-sodium fluoride uptake is consistently observed within the culprit plaque [6] (Fig. 10.1). In patients with stable disease, there is increased ^{18}F-sodium fluoride uptake in plaques with morphologically high risk features which reflects the increased microcalcification, which suggests clinical instability [6] (Fig. 10.2). Whilst provisional data suggest ^{18}F-sodium fluoride positron emission tomography-computed tomography is a potentially valuable tool in cardiovascular risk stratification, the question that remains to be answered is can ^{18}F-sodium fluoride signals provide additional risk prediction beyond clinical risk factor scores, blood biomarkers, and anatomic imaging? This is currently being addressed by the ongoing perspective PRE^{18}FFIR trial (NCT02278211).

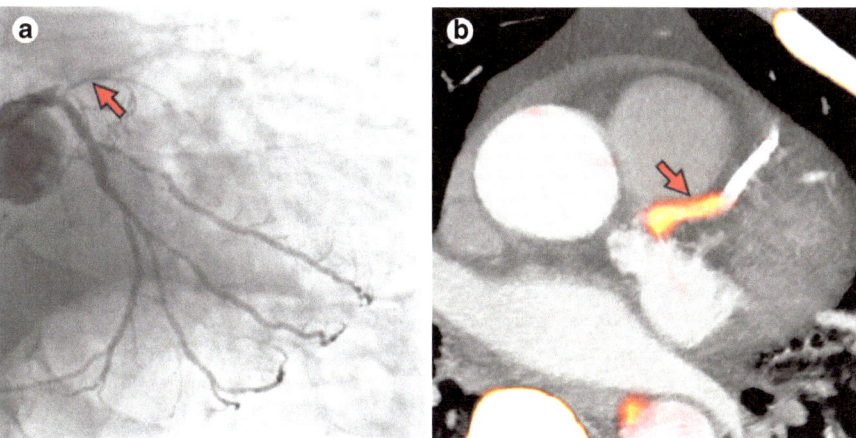

Fig. 10.1 (**a**) Proximal occlusion (*red arrow*) of the left anterior descending artery on invasive coronary angiography and (**b**) intense focal ^{18}F-fluoride [^{18}F-NaF, tissue-to-background ratios, culprit 2·27 versus reference segment 1·09 (108% increase)] uptake (*yellow-red*) at the site of the culprit plaque (*red arrow*) on the combined positron emission and computed tomogram (PET/CT). Adapted from Joshi et al. [6]. [Creative Commons License]

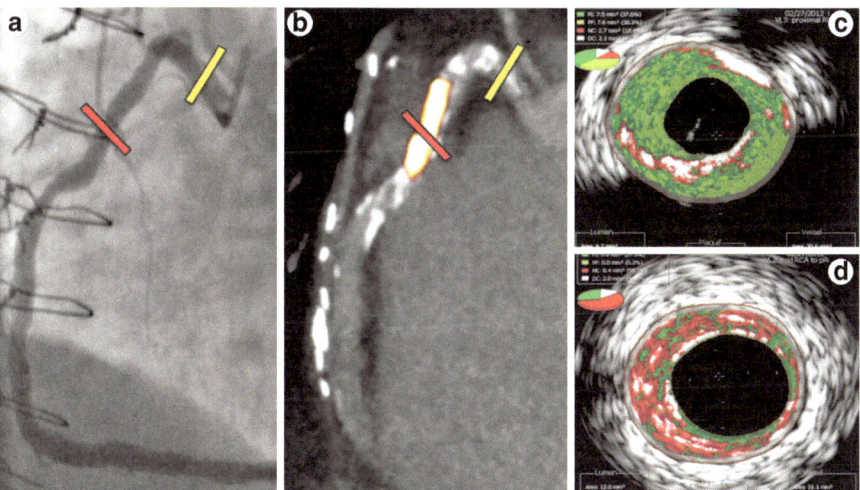

Fig. 10.2 (**a**) Coronary angiogram showing non-obstructive disease in the right coronary artery. Corresponding PET/CT scan (**b**) shows a region of increased ^{18}F-NaF activity (positive lesion, *red line*) in the mid-right coronary artery (tissue-to-background ratio, 3:13) and a region without increased uptake in the proximal vessel (negative lesion, *yellow line*). Radiofrequency intravascular ultrasound shows that the ^{18}F-NaF negative plaque (**c**) is principally composed of fibrous and fibrofatty tissue (*green*) with confluent calcium (*white with acoustic shadow*) but little evidence of necrosis. On the contrary, the ^{18}F-NaF positive plaque (**d**) shows high-risk features such as a large necrotic core (*red*) and microcalcification (*white*). Adapted from Joshi et al. [6]. [Creative Commons License]

10.3   Aortic Stenosis

Aortic stenosis is the most common form of valvular heart disease in the western world [7], which in an aging population represents an increasing healthcare burden. These patients are often elderly with multiple co-morbidities and it can be difficult to allocate symptoms legitimately to the valvular disease, precise evaluation of the severity of aortic stenosis is therefore crucial for patient management and risk strati-fication. In cases with discordant echocardiographic findings, non-invasive imaging modalities capable of quantifying aortic valve calcification can give complementary information and allow prediction of disease progression.

Calcification is believed to be the predominant process driving aortic stenosis progression [8] with hydroxyapatite deposition and leaflet infiltration being the main mechanisms for leaflet restriction and haemodynamic obstruction. The degree of calcification of the aortic valve can be quantitatively and accurately measured on computed tomography and appears to correlate with the haemodynamic severity of aortic stenosis [9, 10].The latest ESC/EACTS Guidelines on valvular heart disease state that in cases of discordant grading, computed tomography calcium scoring (thresholds are 2000 in men and 1250 in women) should be performed as the first-line test [11].

Fused positron emission tomography/computed tomography imaging with ^{18}F-sodium fluoride can assess both the burden of valve calcification demonstrated by the computed tomography calcium score and its activity as measured using ^{18}F-sodium fluoride tracer uptake [12]. Recent clinical studies have shown that ^{18}F-sodium fluoride is taken up by diseased valve and correlates with histological markers of calcification activity [12]. Furthermore, the highest rates of tracer uptake are seen in patient with more severe disease [12] (Fig. 10.3), which might explain why patients on the severe end of the spectrum tend to display greater rates of disease progression. ^{18}F-Sodium fluoride holds promise as a biomarker of disease activity in patients with aortic stenosis and seems to offer additional predictive information over and above the baseline calcium score. The same investigator showed that when patients were recalled for repeat computed tomography calcium scoring at 1 and 2 years, new calcium could be observed in the areas of increased ^{18}F-sodium fluoride activity seen on the baseline scan [12] (Fig. 10.4). Baseline ^{18}F-sodium fluoride uptake therefore predicts disease progression and correlates with adverse cardiovascular events.

There are no medical treatments that can prevent or delay the progression of this disease process. ^{18}F-Sodium fluoride positron emission tomography acts as a marker of disease activity and may be of value in assessing treatment effect of new thera-pies and has been explored as a surrogate end point in ongoing trials looking at the effect of novel drugs on disease activity: the SALTIRE II trial (Study Investigating the Effect of Drugs Used to Treat Osteoporosis on the Progression of Calcific Aortic Stenosis; NCT02132026).

Surgical and interventional valve replacement are currently the only effective treatments for aortic stenosis. The role of ^{18}F-sodium fluoride positron emission tomography/computed tomography in assessing the durability of transcatheter aor-

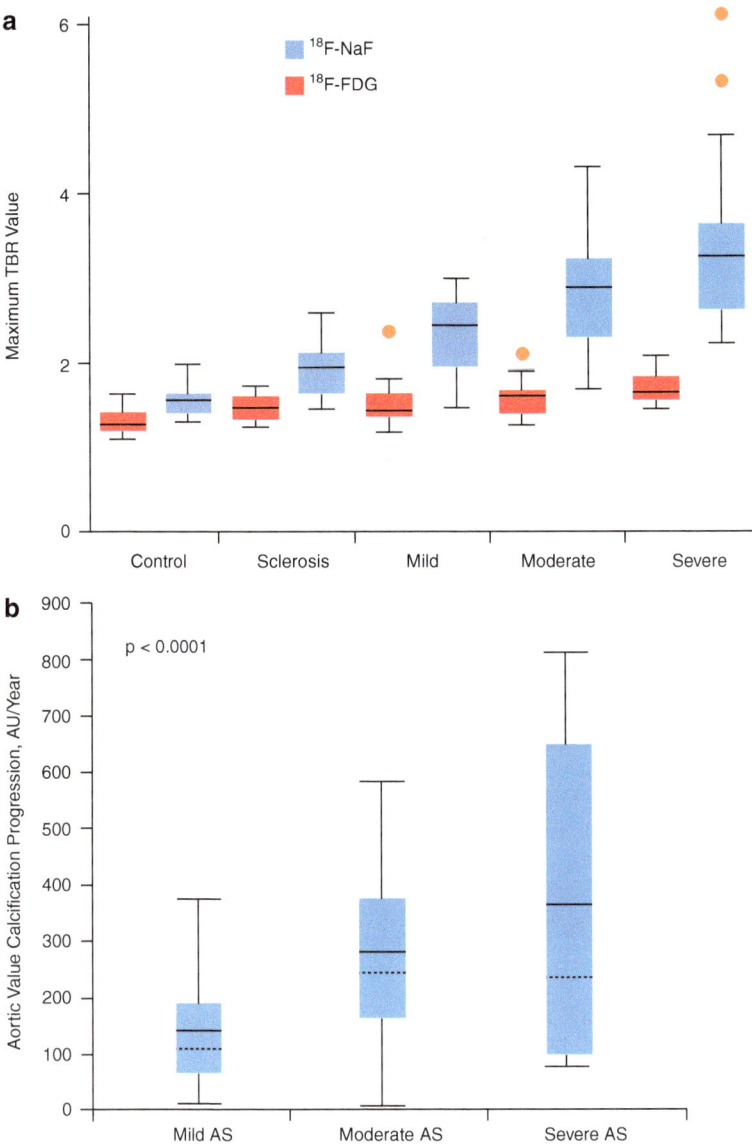

Fig. 10.3 Relationship among baseline disease severity, disease activity and disease progression. (**a**) Studies using PET have demonstrated that calcification activity in the valve (as measured using ^{18}F-fluoride) steadily increases with disease severity. As a consequence, activity is highest in those with the most advanced disease, and a good correlation exists between ^{18}F-fluoride activity and the baseline CT calcium score (79). (**b**) Subsequently, this increased calcification activity appears to translate to more rapid disease progression (as measured by both echocardiography and CT calcium scoring) in patients with the most advanced forms of aortic stenosis (78). *AS* aortic stenosis, *AU* Agatston units, *CT* computed tomography. Adapted from Pawade et al. [8]. [Creative Commons License]

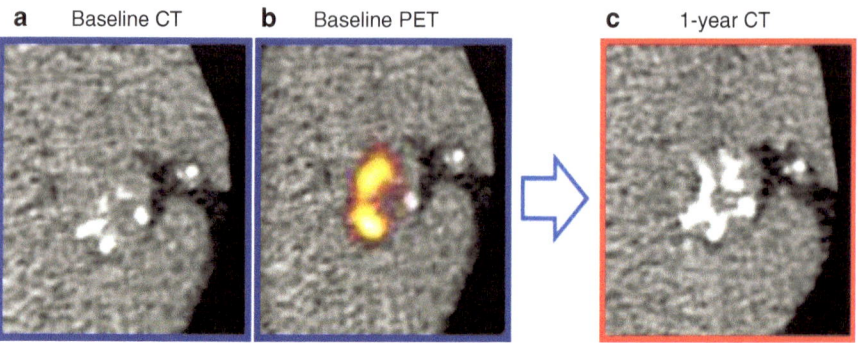

a Baseline CT   **b** Baseline PET   **c** 1-year CT

Fig. 10.4 (**a**)Coaxial short axis views of the aortic valve from a patient with moderate aortic stenosis demonstrated established regions of macrocalcification on baseline computed tomography (CT) scans. (**b**) Fused ^{18}F-fluoride positron emission tomography (PET) and CT showing increased ^{18}F-fluoride activity in the distribution of established calcium deposits and adjacent to regions of calcification. (**c**) At 1 year, novel calcification developed in the regions corresponding to baseline ^{18}F-fluoride activity. Adapted from Chin et al. [13] [Creative Commons License]

tic valve replacement valves is currently under investigation (NCT02304276). Positron emission tomography/magnetic resonance imaging allows simultaneous imaging of calcification activity in the aortic valve using ^{18}F-sodium fluoride alongside the detailed assessments of markers of myocardial decompensation such as midwall late gadolinium enhancement [14] and T1 mapping [15]. One study is looking at using ^{18}F-sodium fluoride positron emission tomography/magnetic resonance imaging to detect early signs of calcification in bioprosthetic valves as an early marker of valve degeneration (NCT03095313) which in the future may help identify patients at risk of rapid valve failure.

10.4 Amyloidosis

Amyloidosis is a well-recognized cause of cardiomyopathy and heart failure, resulting from the inappropriate deposition of insoluble proteins into the myocardium. Cardiac amyloidosis exists in 2 main forms: acquired monoclonal immunoglobulin light-chain (AL) and transthyretin-related (familial and wild-type/senile) amyloid (ATTR). The two forms differ with regards to prognoses and are amenable to different treatment strategies. In patient with ATTR there is evidence that early diagnosis and timely treatment with novel agents (Tafamidis) result in significant improvement in outcomes [16].

Over the last few years, magnetic resonance imaging has been routinely used in the assessment of cardiac amyloid. Amyloid infiltrations typically lead to concentric thickening of the left ventricular walls, which is a relatively non-specific feature. More specific magnetic resonance imaging characteristics of amyloidosis include global subendocardial late gadolinium enhancement, prolonged T1 times and expansion of the extracellular volume. However, these are not able to distinguish between AL and ATRR amyloidosis.

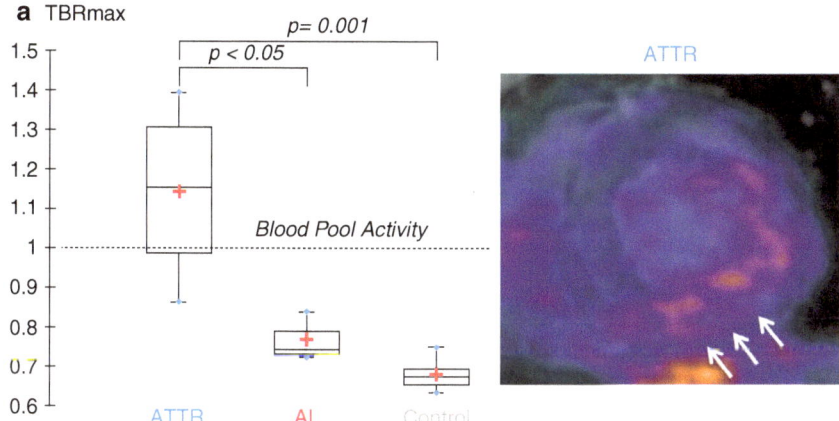

Fig. 10.5 Short-axis hybrid positron emission tomography/magnetic resonance (PET/MR) image demonstrating increased ¹⁸F-sodium fluoride uptake in a patient with transthyretin-related (familial) amyloid (ATTR) colocalizing to areas of late gadolinium enhancement (*white arrows*) in the infero-lateral wall. (**a**) Maximum target-to-background ratio (TBR_{max}) values in patients with ATTR were 48% higher than subjects with acquired monoclonal immunoglobulin light-chain (AL) amyloid and 68% higher than controls, both of whom demonstrated low myocardial uptake, below blood-pool levels (target-to-background ratio . 1.0). Adapted from Trivieri et al. [17] [Creative Commons License]

Hybrid ¹⁸F-sodium fluoride positron emission tomography/magnetic resonance imaging has the potential to do this, with increased ¹⁸F-sodium fluoride uptake observed in areas of ATTR and can effectively differentiate between AL and ATTR [17] (Fig. 10.5). The difference in tracer uptake suggests that the type of amyloid deposits within the myocardium affects local calcium homeostasis. ¹⁸F-Sodium fluoride tracer uptake may be useful for disease monitoring and localizing amyloid deposition in ATTR patients [18]. This is an area of growing interest with ongoing clinical trials (NCT03626584) which should provide a clearer picture of the utility of the ¹⁸F-sodium fluoride positron emission tomography/magnetic resonance imaging in cardiac amyloidosis.

¹⁸F-Sodium fluoride positron emission tomography imaging may be a potential non-invasive tool to differentiate ATTR and AL. Future trials should compare this against the current 'gold standard' of non-invasively differentiating ATTR from AL—99mTc-DPD. ¹⁸F-Sodium fluoride has the advantage of being relatively cheap and readily available, with faster tracer kinetics and imaging times.

10.5   Final Learning Point

The use of ¹⁸F-sodium fluoride positron emission tomography imaging in cardiac disease is currently restricted to the research setting. Given the additional monetary and radiation cost, ¹⁸F-sodium fluoride positron emission tomography is unlikely to replace current gold standard first-line investigations, but has the potential to provide complementary information where the clinical picture is unclear, and has several emerging novel applications that may in the future have clinical utility.

Acknowledgements MD and DEN are supported by the British Heart Foundation (CH/09/002, RE/18/5/34216) and a Wellcome Trust Senior Investigator Award (WT103782AIA).

References

1. O'Malley PG, Taylor AJ, Jackson JL, Doherty TM, Detrano RC. Prognostic value of coronary electron-beam computed tomography for coronary heart disease events in asymptomatic populations. Am J Cardiol. 2000;85:945–8.
2. Dweck MR, et al. Coronary arterial ^{18}F-sodium fluoride uptake: a novel marker of plaque biology. J Am Coll Cardiol. 2012;59:1539–48.
3. Fiz F, et al. ^{18}F-NaF uptake by atherosclerotic plaque on PET/CT imaging: inverse correlation between calcification density and mineral metabolic activity. J Nucl Med. 2015;56:1019–23.
4. de Oliveira-Santos M, et al. Atherosclerotic plaque metabolism in high cardiovascular risk subjects - a subclinical atherosclerosis imaging study with ^{18}F-NaF PET/CT. Atherosclerosis. 2017;260:41–6.
5. Ehara S, Kobayashi Y, Yoshiyama M. Spotty calcification typifies the culprit plaque in patients with acute myocardial infarction: an intravascular ultrasound study. ACC Curr J Rev. 2005;14:39.
6. Joshi NV, et al. ^{18}F-fluoride positron emission tomography for identification of ruptured and high-risk coronary atherosclerotic plaques: a prospective clinical trial. Lancet. 2014;383:705–13.
7. Iung B, et al. A prospective survey of patients with valvular heart disease in Europe: the euro heart survey on Valvular heart disease. Eur Heart J. 2003;24:1231–43.
8. Pawade TA, Newby DE, Dweck MR. Calcification in aortic stenosis. The skeleton key. J Am Coll Cardiol. 2015;66:561–77.
9. Cueff C, et al. Measurement of aortic valve calcification using multislice computed tomography: correlation with haemodynamic severity of aortic stenosis and clinical implication for patients with low ejection fraction. Heart. 2011;97:721–6.
10. Pawade T, et al. Computed tomography aortic valve calcium scoring in patients with aortic stenosis. Circ Cardiovasc Imaging. 2018;11:e007146.
11. Corrigendum to: 2017 ESC/EACTS Guidelines for the management of valvular heart disease. Eur Heart J. 2018;39:1980–1980.
12. Dweck M, et al. ^{18}F-sodium fluoride uptake is a marker of active calcification and disease progression in patients with aortic stenosis. J Am Coll Cardiol. 2013;61:E836.
13. Chin CWL, Pawade TA, Newby DE, et al. Risk stratification in patients with aortic stenosis using novel imaging approaches. Circ Cardiovasc Imaging. 2015;8:e003421.
14. Dweck MR, et al. Midwall fibrosis is an independent predictor of mortality in patients with aortic stenosis. J Am Coll Cardiol. 2011;58:1271–9.
15. Chin CWL, et al. Myocardial fibrosis and cardiac decompensation in aortic stenosis. JACC Cardiovasc Imaging. 2017;10:1320–33.
16. Maurer MS, et al. Tafamidis treatment for patients with transthyretin amyloid cardiomyopathy. N Engl J Med. 2018;379:1007–16. https://doi.org/10.1056/NEJMoa1805689.
17. Trivieri MG, et al. ^{18}F-sodium fluoride PET/MR for the assessment of cardiac amyloidosis. J Am Coll Cardiol. 2016;68:2712–4.
18. Morgenstern R, Yeh R, Castano A, Maurer MS, Bokhari S. [18]Fluorine sodium fluoride positron emission tomography, a potential biomarker of transthyretin cardiac amyloidosis. J Nucl Cardiol. 2017;20:117–9.

¹⁸F-Sodium Fluoride Positron Emission Tomography/Computed Tomography Imaging of the Peripheral Vasculature

11

Maaz B. J. Syed, Jakub Kaczynski, and David E. Newby

Contents

11.1 Introduction

Vascular pathology poses a significant burden on global disease. Vessel calcification is a systemic phenomenon that affects multiple organ beds. Many of the processes leading to vascular calcification share immune-mediated pathways [1, 2]. Contemporary investigative techniques obtain excellent images of morphological features within the vascular system. Established anatomical imaging, such as catheter angiography, computed tomography and magnetic resonance imaging, can accurately visualise the lumen [3]. Advances in computed tomography and magnetic resonance imaging now allow for the non-invasive detection of certain high-risk plaque features [4, 5]. Ultrasound duplex assesses the flow-limiting potential of stenotic lesions to provide a functional measure of vascular disease. Morphological imaging techniques are the basis of modern vascular imaging.

M. B. J. Syed (✉) · J. Kaczynski · D. E. Newby
British Heart Foundation Department of Cardiovascular Sciences, Queens Medical Research Institute, University of Edinburgh, Edinburgh, UK
e-mail: maaz.syed@ed.ac.uk

© Springer Nature Switzerland AG 2020
K. Kairemo, H. A. Macapinlac (eds.), *Sodium Fluoride PET/CT in Clinical Use*,
Clinicians' Guides to Radionuclide Hybrid Imaging,
https://doi.org/10.1007/978-3-030-23577-2_11

Metabolic imaging of the vascular system adds a new perspective to traditional anatomical imaging techniques. Using specially designed radiotracers, we can detect distinct disease processes within the arterial wall. This information allows the early detection of disease before structural changes have manifested. ^{18}F-Sodium fluoride is increasingly being recognised as a radiotracer that can detect arterial wall disease and improve our ability to stratify cardiovascular risk.

11.2   Microcalcification in the Vascular System

Vascular calcification is the product of ongoing metabolic activity within the arterial wall [6]. The formation of visible calcified plaque is a relatively late manifestation of this metabolic activity. ^{18}F-Sodium fluoride binds to exposed hydroxyapatite crystals. These are deposited as the initial building blocks of vascular calcium and later trapped within established plaque [7]. Within the arterial wall, the expression of hydroxyapatite crystals represents intense biological activity that often involves foci of cellular necrosis [8]. This microcalcification occurs at a far smaller scale than the resolution of established imaging techniques.

Positron emission tomography can image the pattern of ^{18}F-sodium fluoride binding within vascular tissue. It is often combined with computed tomography or magnetic resonance imaging to provide anatomical context. A combination of anatomical and metabolic imaging provides a more comprehensive assessment of vascular beds. Whereas computed tomography or magnetic resonance imaging can detect established anatomical changes, ^{18}F-sodium fluoride informs on the biological activity preceding these morphological signs.

11.3   ^{18}F-Sodium Fluoride in the Peripheral Vascular System

11.3.1   Aortic Disease

Diseased aorta undergoes marked architectural and cellular changes in response to hypertension [9], dyslipidaemia [10], smoking [11] and other cardiovascular risk factors. Aortic remodelling involves necrosis of vascular smooth muscle cells, thinning of the medial layer and calcification of elastin fibres [12]. Hypertension causes the endothelium to become permeable to macrophages, which further disrupt the extracellular scaffold of the aortic media through the production of numerous cytokines and matrix metalloproteinases [13, 14]. Consequently, the aorta loses its elasticity and becomes stiff [15]. The net effect is a positive feedback loop of hypertension-driven cellular necrosis within the aortic wall and loss of structural stability. This is accompanied with intense microcalcification.

[18]F-Sodium fluoride can detect aortic microcalcification with high sensitivity [16]. Individuals with no apparent morphological changes in the aorta still exhibit fluoride binding [17]. ^{18}F-Sodium fluoride uptake correlates strongly with established risk scoring systems independent of calcified plaque burden [17, 18]. Established aortic

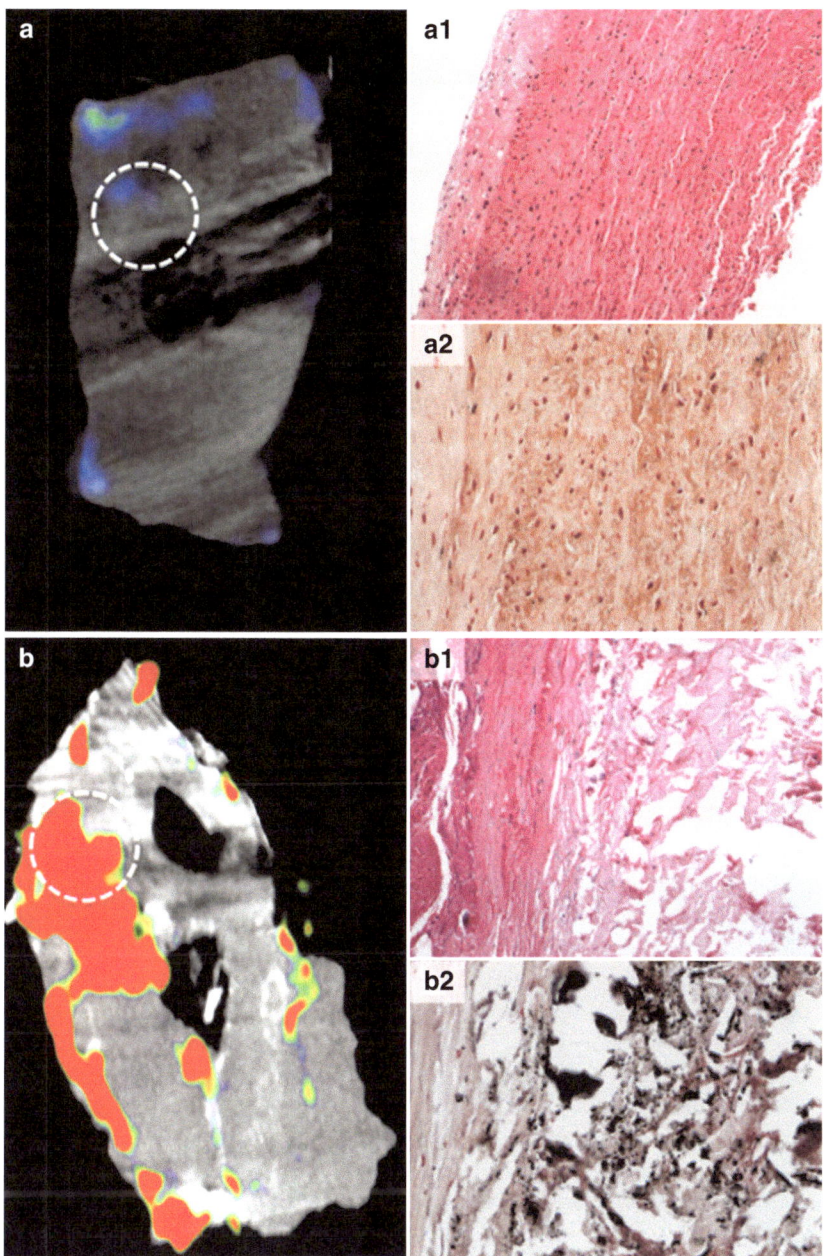

Fig. 11.1 Correlation of histology with micro-positron emission tomography and computed tomography of abdominal aortic tissue. Ex vivo micro-positron emission tomography and computed tomography (*left*) and histology (*right*) of aortic wall excised (**a**) at post mortem in a patient without an aneurysm and (**b**) during open abdominal aortic aneurysm repair. Regions of interest (*dashed circle*) of ¹⁸F-sodium fluoride (¹⁸F-NaF) uptake demonstrate atheromatous disease with necrosis (haematoxylin and eosin stain, magnification ×100; *b1*) and calcification (*black*, Von Kossa stain, magnification ×200; *b2*) in the aortic aneurysm tissue that is not apparent in control aorta (*a1*, *a2*). Adapted from Forsythe et al. [22] [Creative Commons License]

calcification does not improve event prediction beyond coronary calcium scores [19, 20]. ^{18}F-Sodium fluoride detects microcalcification related to increased metabolic activity and holds the promise to be a more sensitive prognostic marker.

The Sodium Fluoride in Abdominal Aortic Aneurysms (SoFIA[3]) study demonstrated increased ^{18}F-sodium fluoride binding throughout the aorta in individuals with aneurysmal disease [21]. Histological analysis of aneurysmal tissue confirmed colocalisation of microcalcification in diseased segments (Fig. 11.1). Interestingly, the study showed marked heterogeneity in the pattern of ^{18}F-sodium fluoride binding suggesting non-uniform microcalcification in aortic aneurysms [22]. These areas of ^{18}F-sodium fluoride binding were separate from regions of established calcified plaque (Fig. 11.2). The SoFIA[3] trial provided valuable insight into the biological mechanisms leading to aneurysmal progression. Aneurysms with the highest uptake of ^{18}F-sodium fluoride demonstrated the fastest rates of growth [22]. This was independent of initial aortic diameter—the traditional morphological parameter used to stratify the risk of aortic rupture.

Histological studies demonstrate cellular necrosis and microcalcification in aortopathies such as acute aortic syndrome and connective tissue disorders [23, 24]. In-house unpublished data suggest that ^{18}F-sodium fluoride binds to these diseased aortic states with a high affinity. The prognostic value of ^{18}F-sodium fluoride positron emission tomography/computed tomography in other aortopathies is the subject of ongoing investigation.

11.3.1.1 Carotid Artery Disease

The identification of culprit plaque represents a key goal in carotid artery imaging. An array of non-invasive imaging techniques, including ultrasound, computed tomography and magnetic resonance imaging, can detect a wide spectrum of complementary high-risk characteristics. However, no single modality can reliably identify vulnerable plaques associated with future stroke development [25, 26]. Substantial histological data suggests that specific plaque components identify patients at high risk for future ipsilateral stroke and cardiovascular events [26, 27]. Culprit carotid plaques exhibit upregulated inflammatory pathways and have increased macrophage infiltration [28]. The lipid rich core is a pool of necrotic material containing remnants of vascular smooth muscle cells that express pro-calcifying receptors on their surface [29]. Consequently, vulnerable plaques are likely to contain microcalcification.

There is a need to look beyond the traditional paradigm of anatomical imaging and obtain information on the arterial wall composition [30]. Alternative non-invasive molecular imaging strategies target not only in vivo carotid morphology

Fig. 11.2 Positron emission tomographic and computed tomographic images of abdominal aortic aneurysms. (**a**) Structural image of computed tomographic angiography, (**b**) ^{18}F-sodium fluoride uptake on positron emission tomography and (**c**) fused positron emission tomographic–computed tomographic images colocalising ^{18}F-sodium fluoride uptake with the skeleton and abdominal aortic aneurysm. Adapted from Forsythe et al. [22] [Creative Commons License]

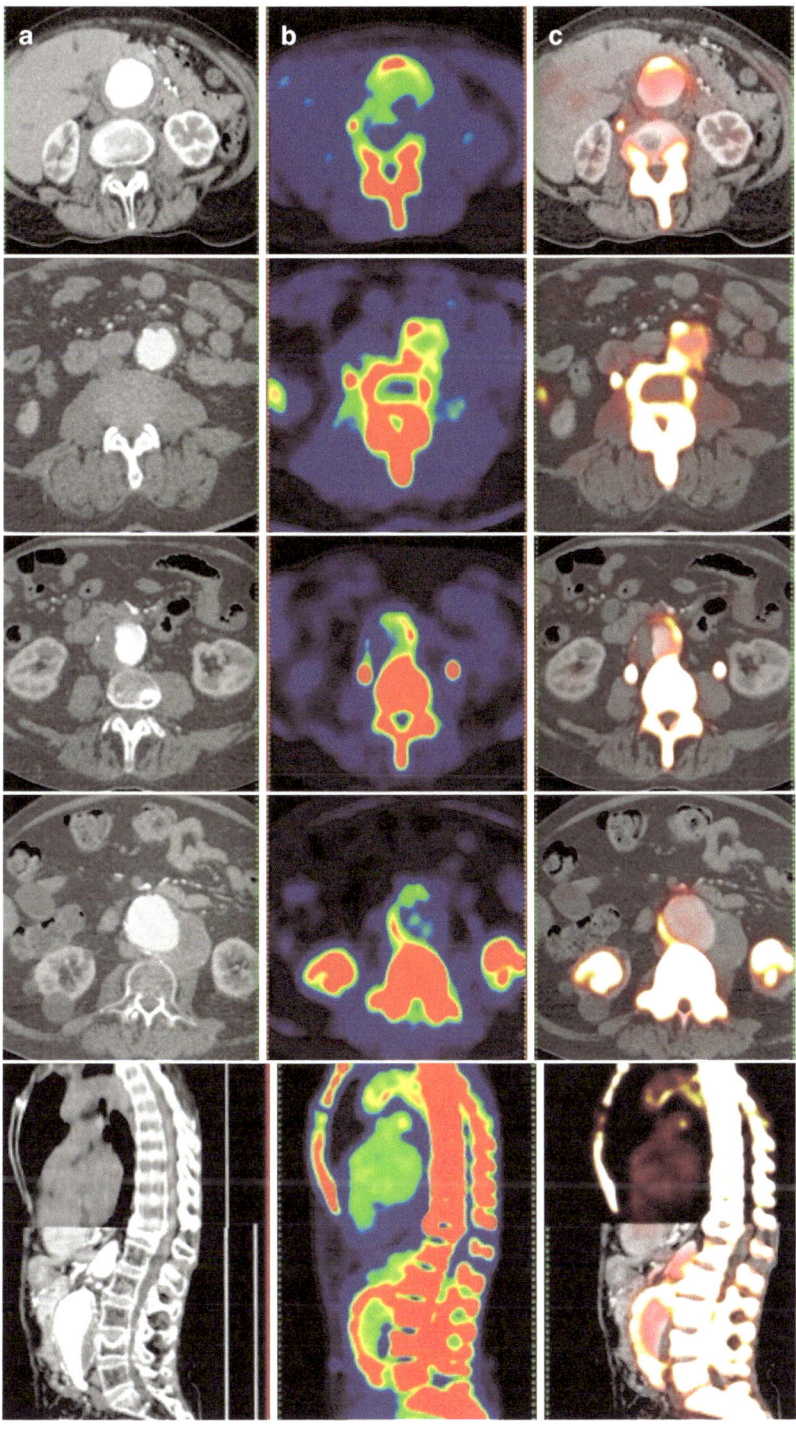

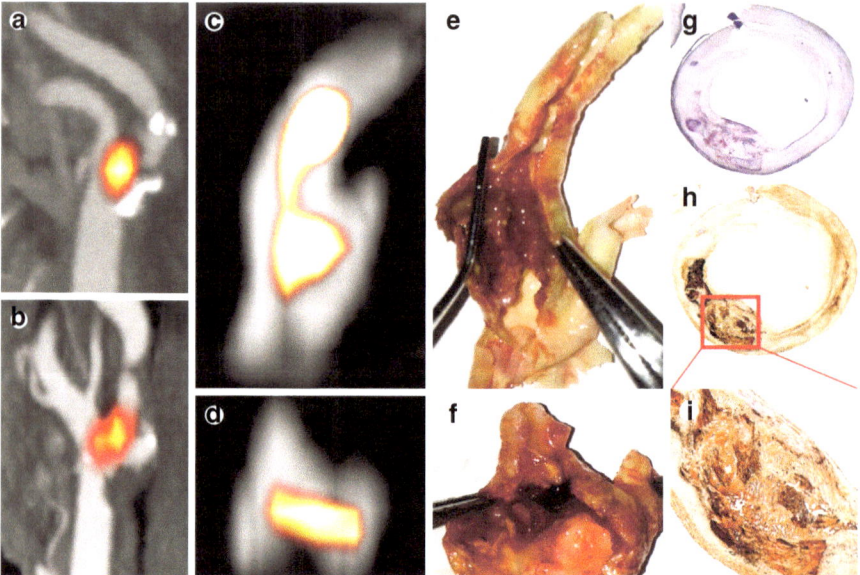

Fig. 11.3 Carotid ^{18}F-NaF uptake and carotid plaque rupture. In vivo (**a** and **b**) and ex vivo (**c** and **d**) positron emission and computed tomograms showing colocalisation of ^{18}F-fluoride (^{18}F-NaF) uptake (yellow–orange) to the site of plaque rupture with adherent thrombus on excised carotid endarterectomy tissue (**e** and **f**). Histology of the ^{18}F-NaF-positive region shows a large necrotic core (Movat's pentachrome, magnification ×4, G), within which increased staining for tissue non-specific alkaline phosphatase can be seen as a marker of calcification activity on immunohisto-chemistry (magnification ×4, **h**; magnification ×10, **i**). Adapted from Joshi et al. [28] [Creative Commons License]

but also plaque biology and disease activity. ^{18}F-Sodium fluoride offers a non-invasive alternative to detect carotid artery microcalcification (Fig. 11.3). It is able to detect metabolic activity in culprit atherosclerotic plaques with a greater accuracy than ^{18}F-fluorodeoxyglucose [31, 32]. Histological and clinical carotid plaque data show high ^{18}F-sodium fluoride uptake localising to areas of plaque rupture in patients with carotid stenosis and recent neurovascular symptoms [31, 33]. Moreover, the tracer is able to discriminate between culprit versus non-culprit plaques (Figs. 11.1 and 11.2). ^{18}F-Sodium fluoride uptake is also associated with high-risk plaque features and with predicted cardiovascular risk (Fig. 11.4).

11.3.1.2   Peripheral Vascular Disease

Vascular calcification adopts specific morphologies in response to different disease states. Atherosclerosis causes intimal disruption and calcium deposition. In conditions such as diabetes mellitus and renal failure, calcified plaque adopts a transmural concentric shape [34]. Both of these patterns are observed in peripheral vessels [35].

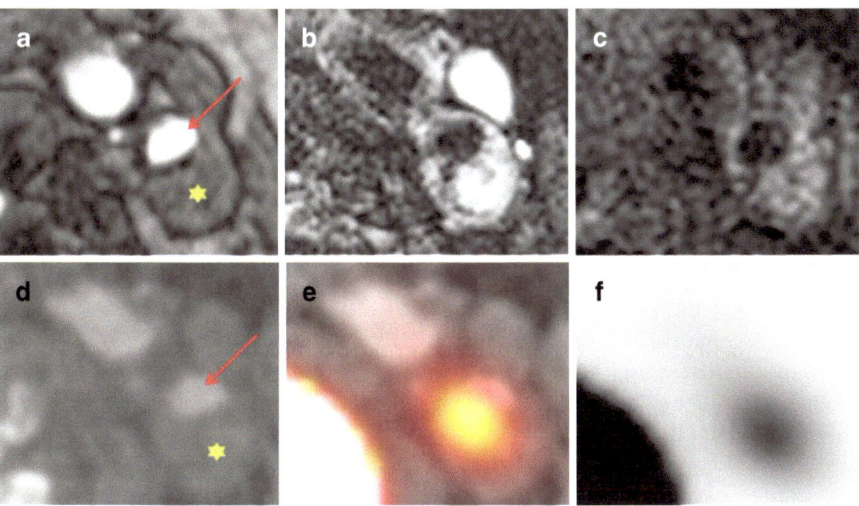

Fig. 11.4 Symptomatic carotid plaque on MRA (3T) and 18F-fluoride positron emission tomography/computed tomography. The *red arrow* denotes the lumen of the ICA, and the *yellow star* denotes culprit haemorrhagic plaque with intense 18F-fluoride uptake. (**a**) Axial time-of-flight MR angiogram. (**b**) T2-weighted image. (**c**) T1-weighted image. (**d**) Computed tomography carotid angiogram. (**e**) Fused positron emission tomography–computed tomography. (**f**) [18F]-Fluoride positron emission tomography. Adapted from Vesey et al. [33] [Creative Commons License]

18F-Sodium fluoride binds to areas of microcalcification in the lower limbs [36]. Fluoride uptake in femoral plaque correlates strongly with dense macrophage infiltration and active inflammation [37]. This is particularly true compared to established radiotracers such as 18F-fluorodeoxyglucose. Clinical studies reveal that 18F-sodium fluoride positron emission tomography/computed tomography of the lower limb arteries reflects the global burden of calcification within the arterial tree and correlates strongly with established cardiovascular risk factors [36]. The impact of these findings to predict peripheral vascular disease progression remains to be validated.

11.4   Improving Risk Stratification

There is a need to go beyond the morphological analysis of vessels alone [38]. Whereas conventional imaging simply identifies morphological changes, 18F-sodium fluoride positron emission tomography/computed tomography detects active disease processes before the vessel exhibits phenotypical change. Combining 18F-sodium fluoride positron emission tomography/computed tomography provides unique insight into the dynamic metabolic state of arterial tissue. Indeed, it can improve our ability to predict aggressive disease progression in at-risk individuals.

Abdominal aortic aneurysms, for instance, may remain dormant for long periods of time. Conversely, some aneurysms grow at an alarming rate. This is associated with an increased risk of aortic rupture. The SOFIA[3] trial shows that ^{18}F-sodium fluoride can detect microcalcification in the aortic wall. Importantly, it was able to predict aortic expansion of small aneurysms before any morphological changes had manifested [22]. The assessment of metabolic activity within the aortic wall represents a fundamentally different perspective on our ability to predict aortic vulnerability.

The current approach to image carotid artery plaque relies predominantly on the detection of internal carotid artery stenosis. However, a significant number of nonstenotic lesions are at risk of plaque rupture. Conversely, a large number of interventions are required to prevent a single episode of recurrent CVA [39]. This suggests that the vast majority of stenosed carotid artery plaques are quiescent. ^{18}F-Sodium fluoride provides a tool to detect high-risk molecular features within carotid atherosclerosis beyond the resolution of computed tomography or ultrasound alone. The prognostic value of carotid artery plaque in conjunction with other high-risk imaging features is the focus of ongoing research.

11.5   Conclusion

Microcalcification in the vascular system is a marker of intense biological activity and reflects areas of focal necrosis within tissue beds. ^{18}F-Sodium fluoride positron emission tomography/computed tomography can detect the deposition of microcalcification accurately in the carotid, aortic and peripheral arteries. Here, ^{18}F-sodium fluoride binding localises to diseased arterial tissue. These findings have been confirmed in histological and clinical studies.

A combination of anatomical and molecular imaging provides unique insight into immune-mediated processes affecting the arterial tree. Understanding these mechanisms allows us to use ^{18}F-sodium fluoride positron emission tomography/ computed tomography to detect disease at a far earlier stage. Traditional imaging modalities can accurately determine vessel morphology and the pattern of calcified plaque. ^{18}F-Sodium fluoride positron emission tomography informs on the biological activity within the arterial wall. Together, ^{18}F-sodium fluoride positron emission tomography/computed tomography promises to improve the risk stratification for specific and general cardiovascular disease progression.

References

1. Teague HL, Ahlman MA, Alavi A, Wagner DD, Lichtman AH, Nahrendorf M, et al. Unraveling vascular inflammation: from immunology to imaging. J Am Coll Cardiol. 2017;70(11):1403–12.
2. Fuery MA, Liang L, Kaplan FS, Mohler ER. Vascular ossification: pathology, mechanisms, and clinical implications. Bone [Internet]. 2017 [cited 2017 Dec 11]. http://www.sciencedirect. com/science/article/pii/S8756328217302326

3. Doris M, Newby DE. Coronary computed tomography angiography as a diagnostic and prognostic tool: perspectives from the SCOT-HEART trial. Curr Cardiol Rep. 2016;18:18.
4. Maurovich-Horvat P, Ferencik M, Voros S, Merkely B, Hoffmann U. Comprehensive plaque assessment by coronary computed tomography angiography. Nat Rev Cardiol. 2014;11(7):390–402.
5. Robson PM, Dey D, Newby DE, Berman D, Li D, Fayad ZA, et al. MR/PET imaging of the cardiovascular system. JACC Cardiovasc Imaging. 2017;10(10):1165–79.
6. Caffarelli C, Montagnani A, Nuti R, Gonnelli S. Bisphosphonates, atherosclerosis and vascular calcification: update and systematic review of clinical studies. Clin Interv Aging. 2017;12:1819–28.
7. Hirsch D, Azoury R, Sarig S, Kruth HS. Colocalization of cholesterol and hydroxyapatite in human atherosclerotic lesions. Calcif Tissue Int. 1993;52(2):94–8.
8. Bentzon JF, Otsuka F, Virmani R, Falk E. Mechanisms of plaque formation and rupture. Circ Res. 2014;114(12):1852–66.
9. Malek AM, Alper SL, Izumo S. Hemodynamic shear stress and its role in atherosclerosis. JAMA. 1999;282(21):2035–42.
10. Ouchi N, Kihara S, Funahashi T, Matsuzawa Y, Walsh K. Obesity, adiponectin and vascular inflammatory disease. Curr Opin Lipidol. 2003;14(6):561–6.
11. Venkatasubramanian S, Noh RM, Daga S, Langrish JP, Mills NL, Waterhouse BR, et al. Effects of the small molecule SIRT1 activator, SRT2104 on arterial stiffness in otherwise healthy cigarette smokers and subjects with type 2 diabetes mellitus. Open Heart. 2016;3(1):e000402.
12. Proudfoot D, Skepper JN, Hegyi L, Bennett MR, Shanahan CM, Weissberg PL. Apoptosis regulates human vascular calcification in vitro: evidence for initiation of vascular calcification by apoptotic bodies. Circ Res. 2000;87(11):1055–62.
13. Aghagolzadeh P, Bachtler M, Bijarnia R, Jackson C, Smith ER, Odermatt A, et al. Calcification of vascular smooth muscle cells is induced by secondary calciprotein particles and enhanced by tumor necrosis factor-α. Atherosclerosis. 2016;251:404–14.
14. Durham AL, Speer MY, Scatena M, Giachelli CM, Shanahan CM. Role of smooth muscle cells in vascular calcification: implications in atherosclerosis and arterial stiffness. Cardiovasc Res. 2018;114(4):590–600.
15. Barrett HE, Cunnane EM, Hidayat H, O'Brien JM, Moloney MA, Kavanagh EG, et al. On the influence of wall calcification and intraluminal thrombus on prediction of abdominal aortic aneurysm rupture. J Vasc Surg. 2018;67(4):1234–1246.e2.
16. Dweck MR, Jenkins WSA, Vesey AT, Pringle MAH, Chin CWL, Malley TS, et al. ¹⁸F-sodium fluoride uptake is a marker of active calcification and disease progression in patients with aortic stenosis. Circ Cardiovasc Imaging. 2014;7(2):371–8.
17. Dweck MR, Chow MWL, Joshi NV, Williams MC, Jones C, Fletcher AM, et al. Coronary arterial ¹⁸F-sodium fluoride uptake: a novel marker of plaque biology. J Am Coll Cardiol. 2012;59(17):1539–48.
18. Blomberg BA, de Jong PA, Thomassen A, Lam MGE, Vach W, Olsen MH, et al. Thoracic aorta calcification but not inflammation is associated with increased cardiovascular disease risk: results of the CAMONA study. Eur J Nucl Med Mol Imaging. 2017;44(2):249–58.
19. Kim J, Budoff MJ, Nasir K, Wong ND, Yeboah J, Al-Mallah MH, et al. Thoracic aortic calcium, cardiovascular disease events, and all-cause mortality in asymptomatic individuals with zero coronary calcium: the multi-ethnic study of atherosclerosis (MESA). Atherosclerosis. 2017;1:1–8.
20. Hoffmann U, Massaro JM, D'Agostino RB, Kathiresan S, Fox CS, O'Donnell CJ. Cardiovascular event prediction and risk reclassification by coronary, aortic, and valvular calcification in the Framingham heart study. J Am Heart Assoc [Internet]. 2016 [cited 2018 Aug 29];5(2). https://www.ncbi.nlm.nih.gov/pmc/articles/PMC4802453/
21. Forsythe RO. Microcalcification predicts abdominal aortic aneurysm expansion and repair: the ¹⁸F-sodium fluoride imaging in abdominal aortic aneurysms (SoFIA3) study. J Vasc Surg. 2017;65(6):24S–5S.

22. Forsythe RO, Dweck MR, McBride OMB, Vesey AT, Semple SI, Shah ASV, et al. ^{18}F–sodium fluoride uptake in abdominal aortic aneurysms: the SoFIA3 study. J Am Coll Cardiol. 2018;71(5):513–23.

23. Wanga S, Hibender S, Ridwan Y, van Roomen C, Vos M, van der Made I, et al. Aortic microcalcification is associated with elastin fragmentation in Marfan syndrome: microcalcification and elastin fragmentation in Marfan syndrome. J Pathol. 2017;243(3):294–306.

24. Ladich E, Yahagi K, Romero ME, Virmani R. Vascular diseases: aortitis, aortic aneurysms, and vascular calcification. Cardiovasc Pathol. 2016;25(5):432–41.

25. Howard DP, van Lammeren GW, Rothwell PM, Redgrave JN, Moll FL, de Vries J-PPM, et al. Symptomatic carotid atherosclerotic disease: correlations between plaque composition and ipsilateral stroke risk. Stroke. 2015;46(1):182–9.

26. Huibers A, de Borst GJ, Wan S, Kennedy F, Giannopoulos A, Moll FL, et al. Non-invasive carotid artery imaging to identify the vulnerable plaque: current status and future goals. Eur J Vasc Endovasc Surg. 2015;50(5):563–72.

27. den Hartog AG, Bovens SM, Koning W, Hendrikse J, Luijten PR, Moll FL, et al. Current status of clinical magnetic resonance imaging for plaque characterisation in patients with carotid artery stenosis. Eur J Vasc Endovasc Surg. 2013;45(1):7–21.

28. Joshi NV, Vesey AT, Williams MC, Shah ASV, Calvert PA, Craighead FHM, et al. ^{18}F-fluoride positron emission tomography for identification of ruptured and high-risk coronary atherosclerotic plaques: a prospective clinical trial. Lancet. 2014;383(9918):705–13.

29. Clarke MCH, Littlewood TD, Figg N, Maguire JJ, Davenport AP, Goddard M, et al. Chronic apoptosis of vascular smooth muscle cells accelerates atherosclerosis and promotes calcification and medial degeneration. Circ Res. 2008;102(12):1529–38.

30. Oliver TB, Lammie GA, Wright AR, Wardlaw J, Patel SG, Peek R, et al. Atherosclerotic plaque at the carotid bifurcation: computed tomography angiographic appearance with histopathologic correlation. AJNR Am J Neuroradiol. 1999;20(5):897–901.

31. Vesey AT, Jenkins WSA, Irkle A, Moss A, Sng G, Forsythe RO, et al. ^{18}F-fluoride and ^{18}F-Fluorodeoxyglucose positron emission tomography after transient ischemic attack or minor ischemic stroke: case–control study. Circ Cardiovasc Imaging. 2017;10(3):e004976.

32. Irkle A, Vesey AT, Lewis DY, Skepper JN, Bird JLE, Dweck MR, et al. Identifying active vascular microcalcification by [(18)]F-sodium fluoride positron emission tomography. Nat Commun. 2015;6:7495.

33. Vesey AT, Dweck MR, Fayad ZA. Utility of combining PET and MR imaging of carotid plaque. Neuroimaging Clin N Am. 2016;26(1):55–68.

34. Moe SM, Chen NX. Mechanisms of vascular calcification in chronic kidney disease. J Am Soc Nephrol. 2008;19(2):213–6.

35. Abedin M, Tintut Y, Demer LL. Vascular calcification: mechanisms and clinical ramifications. Arterioscler Thromb Vasc Biol. 2004;24(7):1161–70.

36. Janssen T, Bannas P, Herrmann J, Veldhoen S, Busch JD, Treszl A, et al. Association of linear ^{18}F-sodium fluoride accumulation in femoral arteries as a measure of diffuse calcification with cardiovascular risk factors: a PET/computed tomography study. J Nucl Cardiol. 2013;20(4):569–77.

37. Stacy MR, Sinusas AJ. Novel applications of radionuclide imaging in peripheral vascular disease. Cardiol Clin. 2016;34(1):167–77.

38. Forsythe RO, Newby DE, Robson JMJ. Monitoring the biological activity of abdominal aortic aneurysms beyond ultrasound. Heart. 2016;102(11):817–24.

39. Rothwell P, Eliasziw M, Gutnikov S, Fox A, Taylor D, Mayberg M, et al. Analysis of pooled data from the randomised controlled trials of endarterectomy for symptomatic carotid stenosis. Lancet. 2003;361(9352):107–16.

Correction to: ^{18}F-Fluoride Imaging: Normal Variants and Artifacts

Guofan Xu

Correction to: K. Kairemo, H. A. Macapinlac (eds.), *Sodium Fluoride PET/CT in Clinical Use*, Clinicians' Guides to Radionuclide Hybrid Imaging, https://doi.org/10.1007/978-3-030-23577-2_2

Chapter 2: A significant portion of the illustration material in this chapter was originally published by Dr. Ismet Sarikaya et al, Normal bone and soft tissue distribution of fluorine-18-sodium fluoride and artifacts on 18F-NaF PET/CT bone scan: a pictorial review. Nuclear Medicine Communication 2017, 38:810-819.

The following figures, for which permission was granted, originate from the work of Sarikaya et al.: Figure in 2.2, page 11; Figures a-d in 2.4, page 13; Figures a, b in 2.5, page 14; Figures a-d in 2.6 and a-f in 2.7, page 15.

The updated online version of this chapter can be found at https://doi.org/10.1007/978-3-030-23577-2_2

© Springer Nature Switzerland AG 2020   C1
K. Kairemo, H. A. Macapinlac (eds.), *Sodium Fluoride PET/CT in Clinical Use*,
Clinicians' Guides to Radionuclide Hybrid Imaging,
https://doi.org/10.1007/978-3-030-23577-2_12

Index

© Springer Nature Switzerland AG 2020

K. Kairemo, H. A. Macapinlac (eds.), *Sodium Fluoride PET/CT in Clinical Use*,
Clinicians' Guides to Radionuclide Hybrid Imaging,
https://doi.org/10.1007/978-3-030-23577-2